D1567324

....
Perspectives of Motor Behavior and Its Neural Basis

Perspectives of Motor Behavior and Its Neural Basis

Editors   *M.-C. Hepp-Reymond*, Zürich
G. Marini, Milan

60 figures and 2 tables, 1997

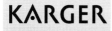

Basel · Freiburg · Paris · London · New York ·
New Delhi · Bangkok · Singapore · Tokyo · Sydney

Library of Congress Cataloging-in-Publication Data
Perspectives of motor behavior and its neural basis / editors, M.-C. Hepp-Reymond, G. Marini.
Includes bibliographical references and index.
1. Locomotion – Regulation.   2. Pyramidal tract.   3. Efferent pathways.   4. Neuromuscular transmission.
5. Motor learning.
I. Hepp-Reymond, M.-C.   II. Marini, Gabriella.
[DNLM: 1. Motor Activity – physiology.   2. Movement – physiology. WE 103 P4672 1997]
QP303.P465   1997
612.7'6 – dc21
ISBN 3-8055-6403-1 (hardcover: alk. paper)

© Copyright 1997 by S. Karger AG, P.O. Box, CH-4009 Basel (Switzerland)
Printed in Switzerland on acid-free paper by Thür AG Offsetdruck, Pratteln
ISBN 3-8055-6403-1

Contents

VII **Preface**

1 **The Pyramidal Tract: Past, Present and Perspective. An Introduction to the Symposium in Honor of Mario Wiesendanger**
Hepp-Reymond, M.-C. (Zürich)

19 **Grasping Objects: The Hand as a Pattern Recognition Device**
Jeannerod, M. (Bron)

33 **Effect of Inactivation of the Hand Representation of the Primary and Supplementary Motor Cortical Areas on Precision Grip Performance in Monkeys**
Rouiller, E.M.; Yu, X.-H.; Tempini, A. (Fribourg)

44 **Balance Control during Movement: Why and How?**
Massion, J. (Marseille)

52 **Quantitative Analysis of Complex Movements**
Pedotti, A. (Milan)

57 **Locomotor Training in Paraplegic Patients**
Dietz, V. (Zürich)

65 **Motor Phenomena during Sleep**
Marini, G. (Milan)

77 **Slow Cortical Potentials Developing Prior to a Self-Paced Voluntary Movement and in a Forewarned Reaction Time Task. A Study in Epileptic Patients with Implanted Electrodes**
Buser, P.; Lamarche, M.; Louvel, J. (Paris)

91 **Transcranial Brain Stimulation for Studying the Human Motor System**
Hess, C.W.; Mathis, J.; Rösler, K.M.; Müri, R. (Bern)

103 **Paths of Discovery in Human Motor Control. A Short Historical Perspective**
Wiesendanger, M. (Bern)

135 **Subject Index**

Preface

This book has arisen from a gathering of selected specialists in the field of motor control who met at a symposium organized by Eric Rouiller at the University of Fribourg (Switzerland), end of 1994, in honor of Mario Wiesendanger on the occasion of his anticipated retirement. Mario Wiesendanger surrendered his chair of Physiology and the directorship of the Institute of Neurophysiology in Fribourg in the spring of 1995 to dedicate himself to the study of neurological patients at the Inselspital in Bern. From an early stage in his career, Wiesendanger devoted his intellectual power to the study of motor control, asking fundamental questions but always keeping in mind the clinical perspective.

The chapters of this book present a large variety of experimental approaches and build an ensemble that should lead to a better understanding of the basic processes involved in the integration of posture and movement for the production of graceful and effective motor acts. It is our belief that, in order to shed light on the complex principles underlying any purposeful behavior, it is absolutely necessary to consider various kinds of methods and technologies, such as electrophysiology, tridimensional representation of movements, electrical and magnetic stimulation techniques, cerebral imaging, and to cover the field from the basic research in animals and human subjects to the clinical applications. The historical aspects treated in the first and last chapters provide a conceptual framework for the more specific contributions.

The first chapter, taking the pyramidal tract as an example of the relation between structure and function, illustrates the development of concepts in motor control research using contributions of Mario Wiesendanger. Two chapters present several features of grasping: from the different types of primate grip patterns to the goal-dependent configuration of the hand and fingers and to the effects of transient inactivation of motor cortical areas on the precision grip performance in monkey. The majority of the chapters deals with human motor control under various perspectives. This includes focusing on: the anticipatory control of balance during movement and the existence of 'kinematic' synergies; basic principles of the tridimensional representation of movements and its application to the analysis of locomotion; features of slow potentials recorded intracortically in patients during various motor strategies, and motor phenomena during sleep with their amazing and still ill-understood pathology. A more clinical chapter presents new approaches to improve the motility of paraplegic patients. Finally, an enlightening review on the use of transcortical magnetic stimulation in the investigation of the normal and pathological motor system is provided. The last chapter by Wiesendanger himself traces the path of the discipline of human motor control from its roots in the last century to contemporary research with its more sophisticated techniques.

At the present time, the 'Masters' seem to be disappearing, due to an accumulation of stimuli, subliminal messages, capillary perceptions, real and virtual experiences. However, an old proverb says: 'If you give a fish to a man, you feed him for one day; if you teach him to fish, you feed him for a lifetime.' This book is dedicated to Mario who taught both of us to fish.

We are grateful to those Institutions which financially supported the realization of this book: University of Zürich, University of Fribourg, Schweizerische Gessellschaft für Physiologie, Centro di Bioingegneria, Fondazione Don Gnocchi e Politecnico di Milano. Our thanks also go to the staff of Karger with whom the making of the book has been most enjoyable.

Marie-Claude Hepp-Reymond
Gabriella Marini

Hepp-Reymond M-C, Marini G (eds): Perspectives of Motor Behavior and Its Neural Basis.
Basel, Karger, 1997, pp 1–18

....

The Pyramidal Tract:
Past, Present and Perspective

An Introduction to the Symposium in Honor of Mario Wiesendanger

Marie-Claude Hepp-Reymond [1]

Brain Research Institute, University of Zürich, Switzerland

The research on the pyramidal tract perfectly illustrates a central question addressed to by science in general and by the neurosciences in particular: the relation between structure and function. Moreover, it is a striking example of the evolution of ideas, of 'beliefs', and of the shifts of interest within scientific domains. The present chapter is an attempt to demonstrate these two points by taking the research field in which Wiesendanger has contributed so much within the last three decades.

The history of the pyramidal tract (PT) is full of correct and incorrect concepts, as far as its function, or functions, is concerned: *'Peu de questions ont suscité autant de travaux que celles qui se rattachent à l'anatomie et à la physiologie des pyramides antérieures'* [1]. This history is closely bound to the history of cerebral localization which, for centuries, has survived successive revolutions in thinking. Presently, cerebral localization coexists with another concept, in appearance contradictory: the parallelism in information processing and motor execution.

This chapter is built in three parts: the distant and near past, the present, and finally, considerations on the future.

The Past

The Distant Past

Much has been written on the history of the PT and the emergence of the relation between this fiber tract, its cortical origin, and the execution of voluntary movements [for reviews, see 2, 3]. The first graphic representation of the PT, a beautiful and intriguing structure, dates from the beginning of the 18th century (fig. 1) and was provided by Pourfour du Petit [4] in 1710. In the same essay, the author also described pertinent clinical and experimental observations in animals on the consequences of PT degeneration on motor behavior.

[1] The author thanks Dr. Roger Lemon and Dr. Kevan Martin for many helpful comments on earlier drafts. Thanks also go to Rita Lindegger for her help with the final editing of the manuscript. The research of the author is supported by the Swiss National Science Foundation (grant 31-39679), the Slack-Gyr and Stanley Thomas Johnson Foundations.

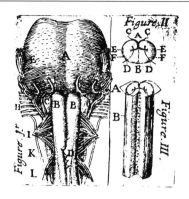

FIGURE I.

Elle réprefente le changement des Fibres Medullaires d'un côté à l'autre.

A   Le *Proceſſus Annullaire.*
B   Les *Corps Piramidaux.*
C   Les *Corps Olivaires.*
D   *La partie inferieure des Corps Piramidaux qui ſe diviſent châcun en*
    trois Manipules de Fibres qui paſſent les unes entre les autres en
    changeant de côté.
E   *La cinquiéme Paire de Nerfs.*
F   *La fixiéme Paire de Nerfs.*
G   *La feptiéme Paire de Nerfs dont la partie dure eſt trop éloignée de*
    la partie molle dans cette Figure.
H   *La huitiéme Paire de Nerfs.*
I   *La neuviéme Paire de Nerfs.*
L   *La dixiéme Paire de Nerfs.*
K   *Le Compagnon de la huitiéme Paire de Nerfs.*

FIGURE II.

Elle réprefente la Moelle de l'Epine coupée en travers.
A   *La diviſion anterieure.*
B   *La diviſion poſterieure.*
C   *Les Nerfs qui ſortent de la partie anterieure de la Moelle.*
D   *Les Nerfs qui ſortent de la partie poſterieure.*
E   *Les Fibres Medullaires tranſverſes.*
F   *Les lignes brunes qui vont de ces Fibres tranſverſes à la partie po-*
    ſterieure.

FIGURE III.

Elle réprefente un morçeau de la Moelle de l'Epine
avec les Fibres Tranſverſes.

A   *La jonction des Nerfs anterieurs avec les poſterieurs.*
B   *La Moelle feparée dans ſa longueur à ſa diviſion poſterieure, au fond*
    de laquelle on voit les Fibres tranſverſes.

Fig. 1. Early 18th century representation of the basal aspect of the brain with bulbar pyramids and their crossing. Original legends of F. Pourfour du Petit, 1710 [4].

A century later, Gall and Spurzheim [5], best known for their extremely popular phrenology, traced the fibers of the PT from the brainstem to the cortex and demonstrated their crossing in the medulla. The 19th century was prosperous in experiments and facts, gained after extirpation of the cortex in diverse vertebrate species. The results were, however, partially contradictory. The anatomical description of the PT from the cortex to the spinal cord dates from this time [6], as well as the convincing correlation between the atrophy of one bulbar pyramid and contralateral hemiparesis following a lesion of the hemisphere on the same side as the shrunken PT [7].

The investigations of Fritsch and Hitzig [8] and of Ferrier [9] finally gave support to the concept of cerebral localizations previously formulated by Paul Broca [10]: '*Je crois au principe des localisations. Je ne puis admettre que la complication des hémisphères cérébraux soit un simple jeu de la nature. … L'existence d'une première localisation une fois admise, le principe des localisations par circonvolutions serait établi*' [p. 339]. With these investigations, the motor cortex was born and the major function of the PT in the control of voluntary movement was established. The origin of the PT was then localized by Sherrington [11] in a cortical region which he named 'cord area'; he thus stressed the close relation between cortex and spinal cord and treated the PT as an 'internuncial system'.

The discovery by Betz [12] of another marvellous structure in search of a function, the giant pyramidal cells in area 4, prompted to restrict the functions of the PT to this area, called motor cortex, and particularly to these large neurons. '*Ich werde sie Riesenpyramidalzellen nennen … Diese Riesenpyramiden sind an den bezeichneten Stellen in jedem menschlichen Gehirne, beim Idioten, beim Chimpanse, beim grauen, braunen, beim kleinen persischen Pavian und beim grünen Affen vorhanden* [p. 580] ... *Diese Zellen besitzen zweifellos alle Attribute sogenannter "motorischer" Zellen und setzen sich ganz bestimmt als Gehirnfasern fort'* [p. 581]. This belief was to last for a long time.

The first half of the 20th century was full of investigations trying to elucidate the mysteries of the PT and of its function: corticospinal connectivity and its characteristics, anatomical data based on degeneration studies, motor deficits after ablation of motor cortex or transection of the bulbar pyramids. Again, some of the results were contradictory and generated many controversies and disputes, in which Walshe [13, 14] has been one of the most eloquent and aggressive representatives.

The Near Past

In 1969, Wiesendanger [15] summarized, in his important review, 'The Pyramidal Tract. Recent Investigations on its Morphology and Function', the state of the knowledge available in the 1960s. He focused mainly on aspects of connectivity, shown by neuroanatomical and electrophysiological techniques. To quote some of the most important ones: (1) Detailed neuroanatomy of the PT with its origin, fiber number and destinations. (2) Electrophysiological properties of identified PT neurons (PTNs). (3) Influence of electrical stimulation of the PT and motor cortex on spinal cord mechanisms, in particular on the primate α-motoneurons [16] and possibly on γ-motoneurons. (4) Sensory input to the pyramidal cells, accounting for the so-called 'relayed pyramidal discharge' [17] and identification of small receptive field on a minority of PTNs [18]. (5) Role of recurrent axons in intracortically shaping the output of the PTNs by recurrent inhibition [19].

Figure 2, taken from Wiesendanger's review, illustrates the anatomofunctional knowledge of this time. A small detail, interesting from the historical point of view, are the cPT, collaterals of the PT, drawn at a time when their existence had not yet been demonstrated, neither in anatomical nor in physiological terms. It was assumed that all the cortico-subcortical projections, identified anatomically on the basis of degeneration, could only be collaterals of the PT fibers: these were required as substrates for the expected internal feedback loops that are indispensable to motor control.

The 1969 review also summarized the first reports on neuronal correlates of voluntary movements: at that time, Evarts [20, 21] had just made his pioneer contributions in awake trained monkeys and had demonstrated the relation of the PTN activity to movement initiation, and to force. Evarts [22] had recently resurrected the central question asked a century earlier by Hughlings Jackson [23] and again by Phillips [24]: Was there evidence from such recordings that the motor cortex represented muscles or movements?

One central preoccupation at the end of the 1960s concerns the deficits induced by lesion of the PT, in particular the fundamental differences between the so-called 'pyramidal syndrome' in patients, characterized by paresis, spasticity, exaggeration of tendon reflexes, depression of cutaneous reflexes and Babinski sign, and the motor deficits observed in monkeys after pyramidotomy. In monkeys, the leading symptom is a flaccid paralysis and, as elegantly shown by Lawrence and Kuypers [25], a major impairment of fractionated finger movements, attributed to the interruption of the corticomotoneuronal (CM) fibers. This publication was very influential in dismissing spasticity as a central effect of the pyramidal syndrome and in focusing the attention on the importance of the hand skill as a primary feature of the PT. However, there was still a lack of quantitative assessment of the deficits and of their recovery over time.

Wiesendanger [15] concluded his review by asking one at this time fundamental question: *'Does the pyramidal tract have unique features,'* or in other words, *'how many of*

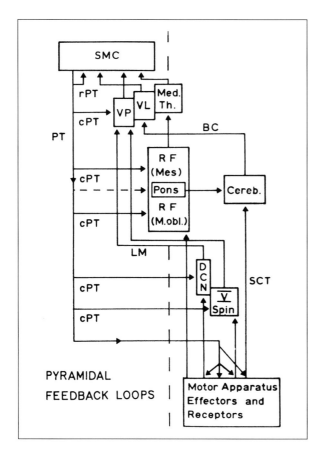

Fig. 2. Diagram of pyramidal feedback connections. The pyramidal fibers give off recurrent collaterals (cPT), collaterals to thalamic nuclei (VP, VL, Med. Th.), the reticular formation (RF) of the mesencephalon (Mes.) and of the lower brain stem (M. obl.), the dorsal column nuclei (DCN), and the spinal trigeminal nucleus (V spin.). The pyramidal fiber terminals influence the motor units and receptors (muscle spindle) and spinal neurons projecting to higher centers, especially to the cerebellum (SCT, Cereb.). All recipients of the collaterals have again connections to the sensorimotor cortex (SMC). BC = Brachium conjunctivum; LM = lemniscus medialis. (From Wiesendanger [15], with permission.)

the mechanisms described are typical or even unique for the pyramidal tract?' [p. 121]. In this context, several observations were intriguing, such as the fact that stimulation of other descending pathways had similar effects on the α- and γ-motoneurons. Another puzzling observation was the motor recovery after pyramidotomy in cats, monkeys, and even in some patients, an observation that is still not completely understood. However, one characteristic is unique to the PT of primates: its CM system. Wiesendanger's 1969 review ended with the hope that subtle and quantitative conditioning methods might yield satisfactory information on the correlates of single neuron mechanisms, and thus provide the information necessary to solve all the contradictions.

In 1969, the 'precision grip story' is already born, and a short time later our first quantitative results come out, exciting and encouraging, but in retrospect meagre. After

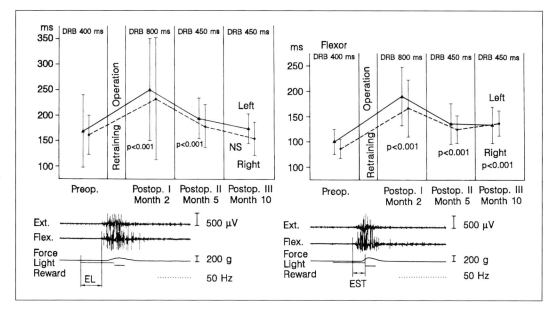

Fig. 3. Above: Specific deficits and partial recovery in a reaction time experiment in one monkey after bilateral pyramidotomy. The monkey had to reach a low force level as fast as possible after the 'go' signal, by compressing a small force transducer between thumb and index finger. Both EMG latency (EL) (left) and EMG summation time (EST) (right) showed significant increase after surgery (Postop. I and II). After 10 months (Postop. III), EL had again reached preoperative values, whereas EST remained increased. Average values of 100–200 trials with SD (vertical bars). —— = Left hand; ---- = right hand. Below: Two examples of single trials with EMG activity in flexors and extensors and force traces. (From Hepp-Reymond [3], with permission.)

complete transection of the PT axons, even after a bilateral one, the monkeys can after a short recovery time exert force between thumb and index finger. The execution is slowed down, and the slowness is irreversible in cases of bilateral pyramidotomy [26]. With time and regular training the monkeys managed to grab food morsels with their fingertips in a Klüver board, and the initial clumsiness disappeared. This observation was confirmed later by Chapman and Wiesendanger [27], who described the strategies used by the animals to compensate for their deficits. These observations which apparently contradicted Lawrence and Kuypers' [25] observations were mainly suggesting that recovery could be enhanced by intensive training, and that the precision grip may not require the same type of control as rapid independent finger movements.

This quantitative assessment of the motor deficits and of the EMG activity, relatively new in 1972, did not add greatly to knowledge as to the function of the PT, when compared to the first careful qualitative observations of Tower [28], but they revealed that the long-term impairment concerns exclusively the execution of the movement, not its initiation (fig. 3).

In 1981, a second review by Wiesendanger [29] again addressed the structure and function of the PT. What happened between 1969 and 1981 to warrant another review on the same subject? The answer is the appearance of a series of new concepts, and a slow but continuous shift of focus. Wiesendanger made important contributions to both directions. The most significant new facts are summarized below:

(1) Firstly, the quantitative motor deficits after pyramidotomy, mentioned above, demonstrated that the PT is necessary but not indispensable for relatively precise finger movements, such as the grip, and for grip force in the macaque monkey [26, 30].

(2) Secondly, the refinement of neuroanatomical techniques and of functional neuro-anatomy. Thanks to intracellular electrophysiology and staining of cell bodies with injection and transport of fluorescent or radioactive substances, it is now clear that the motor cortex contains many neuronal populations with targets such as the striatum, thalamus, red nucleus, precerebellar nuclei such as the lateral reticular nucleus, and dorsal column nuclei. The scheme presented in 1969 has been expanded and modified: the cPTs were erased and replaced by direct cortico-subcortical projections. The proportion of PT axons with collaterals that project to subcortical structures is still a matter of debate and requires more research. This question was addressed by Wiesendanger and co-workers for the lateral reticular nucleus [31] and the corticopontine projections [32]. However it was only with Keizer and Kuypers [33] that the problem of the collaterals could be tackled with the method of double labelling of cell bodies by retrograde transport of different fluorescent substances.

(3) The issue that in my opinion has occupied most scientists interested in the motor system, contributed most publications in human subjects and anesthetized or awake monkeys, and raised many controversies, is the problem of the input-output linkage. The existence of a peripheral sensory input to motor cortex and of a tight input-output linkage with radial organization had been shown by Asanuma [34] first in cats then in monkeys. Moreover, the projection of muscle afferents to the motor cortex, to PTNs, had also been finally established by Wiesendanger [35] after many hot debates [36]. This pyramidal feature requires a function, and the end of the 1970s witnessed interminable discussions on the origin of the components M1, M2 and M3 of a muscle response to a sudden stretch – spinal, supraspinal or cortical –, on the existence of the famous long-loops, the transcortical reflexes, and their putative functional role. All the big names in motor control participated in this fashionable research. First of all is Charles Phillips [37] who formulated the concept of the transcortical loop, and proposed that the increase of cortical activity, which occurred when the movement was resisted by a load, could not be interpreted as an abstract force command, but resulted from a mismatch between intended and actual displacement. Phillips' hypothesis stimulated many investigators: e.g. Conrad et al. [38], Evarts and co-workers [39, 40], Wiesendanger and co-workers [41, 42] and Cheney and Fetz [43] who demonstrated later the participation of CM cells in the transcortical reflexes. The tight relation between the periphery (cutaneous and/or proprioceptive afferences) and the PTNs, according to several authors, should be responsible for the placing reactions that disappear after pyramidotomy, for the grasp reflex, and for the reactions to unexpected perturbations and their partial compensation.

(4) With respect to the CM system itself, electrophysiological and anatomical experimental evidence revealed a spinal branching of single corticospinal axons which diverge to several motoneuronal pools [44, 45]. This intraspinal branching was also supported by Fetz and Cheney [46] in awake monkeys trained to make a flexion-extension movement of the wrist. A new concept was created, the 'muscle field'. This discovery shed new light on the functions of the CM system, which apparently does not consist exclusively of cells projecting to specific muscles but may be implicated in the organization of complex muscular synergies, even involving several spinal segments.

(5) Another essential advance before 1981 was the characterization of the quantitative relations between neuronal activity and motor behavior, in other words the encoding of

movement parameters. Our research on the central control of the precision grip has expanded in this direction and has provided important quantitative data on the neuronal correlates of the rate of force change (dF/dt [47]) and of finely graded constant grip force in identified PT cells and nonidentified motor cortical cells [48]. Neuronal correlates of other variables are also proposed by other groups, and Thach [49] first demonstrated that the activity of single motor cortex neurons can be related to at least three variables, joint position, muscle activity, and direction set.

Against a simple neural coding of force in response to the application of a load, Evarts [50, 51] suggested that the pyramidal neurons in the motor cortex are 'summing points' between central commands and peripheral input in a closed loop system, and that they are mostly active in small controlled movements. Thus, an increase in firing rate in these slow precise movements would be caused by an increase of the peripheral feedback and not by an abstract central command.

(6) Finally, the 'secondary' motor areas, particularly the supplementary motor area (SMA), began to attract some interest. The contemporary knowledge on these areas was presented by Wiesendanger [52] in his chapter of the Handbook of Physiology. He stressed the controversial literature on the function of the premotor cortex and the still poor understanding of the functions of the SMA. The access of the SMA to the spinal cord, considered at that time to be minimal, and its bilateral projections to the precentral cortex suggest that the SMA is hierarchically higher than primary motor cortex. It could be involved in postural adaptations [53] and also is an ideal candidate for gating of proprioceptive afferences in the motor cortex and for exerting some control on transcortical reflexes [54].

The conclusion drawn from this wealth of new information was that: *'The pyramidal tract should be considered as a multicomponent system. Its functions have to be understood not in isolation but in conjunction with inputs and targets'* [29, p. 472]. These sentences opened a wide research program in the years that followed. Among the many issues which remain unsolved, Wiesendanger selected a series of questions, for the majority bound to connectivity: (1) Among the projections of the motor cortex to subcortical targets, which ones are specific and which ones belong to collaterals of corticospinal fibers to the same targets? (2) Does the CM system mainly consist of 'fast' PTNs? This is expected since manual dexterity requires velocity. But what is the role of the 90% 'slow' PTNs? Can a special function be attributed to them? (3) Are the deficits after pyramidotomy mainly due to the interruption of the fast PTNs? (4) What is the function of the PTNs projecting to the ipsilateral spinal cord? (5) What is the role of the PT in postural adaptations? Could the divergence of spinal terminations imply such a role, or is the PT exclusively implicated in distal movements?

The Present

The wind blowing from 1981 to the present is an innovative one: the issues of simple connectivity have become secondary considerations. Although major contributions are still made in neuroanatomy, operational aspects have gained more weight and influence, and occupy the forefront of research. New aspects of motor control flourish, such as 'higher brain functions' [55, 56], and the scientific interest shifts from the neuronal correlates of simple motor parameters to the representation of more abstract and cognitive aspects of movement. Regions outside of the primary motor cortex are much more attractive for modern studies and, among those, the SMA, to use Wiesendanger's [57] words, 'supramotor' area, is particularly popular. From a gating area for peripheral sensory input, it develops into a higher brain area, which should play a central role in movement initiation, a kind of organizing center [58]. Many virgin areas are waiting for an intrepid explorer.

On the basis of some examples chosen among the explosion of facts and new concepts which has taken place in the last 10–15 years, I would like to lead to the present state of knowledge at the end of the 20th century. If one looks for the term 'pyramidal tract' in the index of the recent book of Porter and Lemon [59] on 'Corticospinal Function and Voluntary Movement' one finds: 'see corticospinal tract'. There is no longer a pyramidal tract! What happened to account for such a disappearance?

Multiple Origin of the PT

The inhomogeneity and multifunctional role of the PT, and even of the corticospinal tract, which had been described several times before is now widely confirmed and re-emphazised. The corticospinal tract arises spread from a large number of regions in the frontal cortex, even including the cingulate gyrus (areas 23 and 24) [60]. These multiple motor regions within the frontal lobe contain one or several more or less complete representations of the body, as shown by intracortical microstimulation. The somatotopical organization, even in the primary motor cortex, has lost its simplicity in favor of more complex models with multiple representations of the muscle groups and new types of spatial organization, such as the nested or horseshoe one [61, 62], or multiple body maps, already suggested by Lemon et al. [63] and by Strick and Preston [64].

Are all these regions with direct access to the spinal apparatus equivalent? Do they represent a highly redundant motor cortical control system? Their existence challenges the idea of a simple hierarchical organization with the primary motor cortex as a final major executor of movement [65].

From the anatomical point of view, the connectivity of each area, or subarea, seems to be quite specific. As an example, according to Schell and Strick [66], the SMA receives its major input from the basal ganglia, via the VA and VLo of the thalamus while the motor cortex is mainly the target of the cerebellum over the VPLo (for abbreviations, see legend of fig. 4). However, such a simple dichotomy does not really reflect the anatomical complexity as Wiesendanger and Wiesendanger [67, 68] found by means of transneuronal labelling. They showed that the cerebellum projects to SMA, though to a lesser degree, and that the thalamic subdivisions area X and VLc are regions of convergence of striatal and cerebellar outputs (fig. 4). In fact, a high degree of specific neuroanatomical connectivity seems to be the rule [69].

From the functional point of view, two completely contradictory conclusions can be drawn from the experimental facts: regional specialization with division of labor, or in contrast, striking distribution of function and parallel processing. The first is mainly suggested by specific deficits following lesions in the premotor cortex and SMA [70–72], the second emerges from many investigations on single unit activity in awake trained monkeys, mostly those on the coding of 'simple' movement parameters. The research on neuronal activity in precision grip illustrates the redundancy. Neurons in several cortical areas and subcortical regions discharge during the precision grip task in a manner similar to primary motor cortical neurons [for review, see 3]. In a visuomotor paradigm requiring the production and precise control of successive force steps, no obvious differences in the force-related activity of the neurons in primary motor cortex, premotor cortex, thalamus and globus pallidus were found [73–75]. All the neuronal characteristics tested were represented in each of these structures, and only subtle differences in the relative distribution

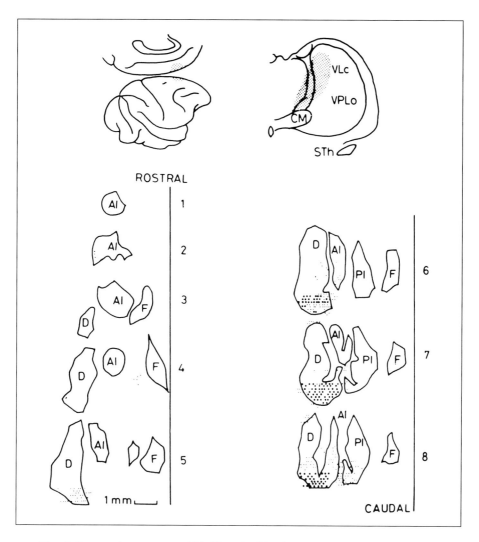

Fig. 4. Retrograde transneuronal labelling of cell bodies in the cerebellar nuclei after injection of WGA-HRP in the rostral SMA. Upper left: Injection site in the SMA. Upper right: Thalamic labelling. Below: Diagrammatic representations of the deep cerebellar nuclei in transverse sections. Small dots represents weakly labelled cells, large dots are cells with relatively dense transcellular labelling. AI = Anterior interposed nucleus; PI = posterior interposed nucleus; D = dentate nucleus; F = fastigial nucleus; VLc, VPLo = thalamic nuclei (ventrolateral caudal and ventroposterolateral, respectively); CM = centromedian nucleus. (From Wiesendanger and Wiesendanger [68], with permission.)

of the various properties in the different regions could be the substrate of some regional specialization. Other groups of investigators using different experimental and behavioral paradigms also reached similar conclusions [76–81]. An extensive discussion of this issue for the frontal cortical areas and for arm and hand movements has been presented by Humphrey and Tanji [82]. Seal et al. [83] also conclude from their and others' findings: *'The differences ... thus seem to be more quantitative than qualitative'* [p. 58].

New Concepts for the Neuronal Correlates

Three new avenues in the neuronal correlates of movement characterize the modern times:

First, the evolution of the research effort from the central control of unidimensional movements to that of bi- or tridimensional movements [84–87]. The movements in the 2- or 3-D space require the coordination of a large number of muscles, taken as a complex synergy, and not only the simple activation of one group of synergists as in previous motor tasks. These investigations demonstrate the multiple representation of movement direction in parietal, motor and premotor areas. The patterns of neuronal activity cannot be simply assigned to one specific muscle or group of synergists. Moreover, the activity of a whole population, as population code or vector, is a better predictor of the movement direction than the firing rate of single neurons. The interpretation of the directional coding though is still a matter of debate and is moving from an abstract internal representation of the cartesian coordinate system [88] to that of a body-centered space in the frontal motor areas after visuomotor transformation in the parietal lobe [89, 90].

The second, and most modern tendency can be summarized by the following quotation which serves as introduction to the book of Evarts et al. [54] 'Neurophysiological Approaches to Higher Brain Functions': *'We would like to step back from the actual mechanisms involved in executing motor commands and from the various servomechanisms or obligatory reflexive mechanisms which operate the motor apparatus. We intend largely to ignore the mechanisms of movement execution and hope to gain better understanding of higher brain function. Our approach is to 'work backwards', to start from the behavior … It is our contention, then, that the study of brain circuits which lie at the basis of higher brain function is possible without a complete analysis of the 'lower' functions'* [p. 2].

This quotation, which may be considered as Evarts' testament, represents a major shift of interest in motor control: from a 'bottom-up' to a 'top-down' approach. The main aim now is to search at the unitary level for the central representation of cognitive processes: attention, intention, sensory and motor sets, motor programs. This view of the brain and of motor control gives a new vigor to the investigation of the motor system and provides new concepts with which the so-called 'association' areas, such as various premotor and parietal areas, can be attacked.

The main proponents and initiators of this new wave are Wise and co-workers [91], who systematically investigate the neuronal correlates of 'motor set' or movement preparation in the premotor cortex, and Tanji and co-workers [92, 93], who mainly try to solve the riddle of the SMA in movement organization, and to disclose its functional specializations as compared to the motor and lateral premotor cortex. Over the last years, paradigms of extreme subtlety and complexity, based on concepts inspired from experimental psychology, have been conceived, in order to dissociate the various factors, as for example the role of different prior instructions [94], or the dissociation between visuomotor and visuospatial information [95] or between intention and attention before movement execution [96]. Our own investigations on the precision grip have also been extended through a more complex protocol. These should lead to a better understanding of the neuronal correlates recorded in the premotor regions, and help to dissociate the simple force coding from the representation of instructions or intention. Under these new conditions, context-dependent force-related activity has been found in the premotor cortex, albeit not exclusively there, since such neurons were also located in the motor cortex [97, and Qi, PhD thesis]. One of the most striking results along this 'top-down' line of research is that of Tanji and Shima [98], who recently were able to demonstrate that neuronal activity in the SMA can represent

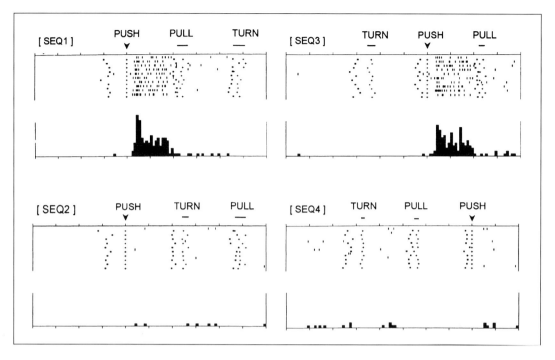

Fig. 5. Selective activity of an SMA cell during a waiting period in between a single combination of two specific movements. This neuron is preferentially active before the 'pull' movement if the previous movement is 'push' (top, SEQ1 and SEQ3), but not if the previous movement is 'turn' (bottom, SEQ2 and SEQ4). Small squares, crosses and triangles denote the times of occurrence of the trigger signal, movement onset and target acquisition. In histograms, discharges over 12 trials are summated. Monkeys were required to place the manipulandum to a neutral position and wait 2.5–4.5 s for the first movement trigger signal. When the monkey performed the first movement, a mechanical device returned the manipulandum to the neutral position. While keeping the manipulandum in this position, the monkey had to wait for 1 s for the second and then for the third movement. (From Tanji and Shima [98], with permission.)

motor sequences in a precise context like a selective activation during the interval between two specific movements, e.g. before a push movement, but only if the next move will be a pull (fig. 5). They even found SMA neurons preferentially active in relation to a particular order of movement guided by memory, without any sensory cues. In this new research trend, the identification of the classes of neurons by antidromic stimulation of the bulbar pyramids or of other subcortical targets, which had been a central preoccupation of earlier studies, is secondary and rarely done, except for very specific questions [99]. The global operation is what matters, and advances in this domain could give material for interesting theoretical modelling.

A third recent move in the exploration of cortical motor functions is taking place under the influence of human motor psychophysics. Investigations of some selected motor behaviors in humans have led to the concept of 'motor invariance', which should correspond to a higher level of motor organization, whose central substrate is still completely unknown. Several observations on the behavioral level have thus stimulated scientists to investigate the neuronal correlates of motor invariances. Three examples are apposite at this point, all concerned with the hand and with grasping function:

(1) The influence of cutaneous inputs in the precision grip and in the regulation of force during grasping objects. Johansson [100] very elegantly demonstrated the presence of a strong invariance in the automatic control of manipulative tasks. The control of load and grip forces appears to be subjected to constraints which have the goal of maintaining a constant grip force/load force ratio with an inbuilt safety margin. These systematic and very convincing observations have led Smith and co-workers to investigate the neuronal correlates of this behavior in the cerebellum and motor cortex [101]: They uncovered groups of neurons whose activity is exquisitely modulated by the surface texture or even more by the surface friction and could serve as modulators of the muscle commands in the grip force regulation [102].

(2) The organization of reaching and grasping under visual control, with the emergence of a 'goal-directed invariance', that is, the coordinated kinematics of the transport of arm and wrist and of the finger opening and closing [103]. The existence of two parallel motor programs have been suggested, and demonstrated experimentally or clinically, and a close interaction between both has been hypothesized [Jeannerod, chap. 2]. Neuronal correlates for grasping and reaching have now been found in the inferior and superior parietal lobules respectively, which form specialized networks with specific premotor regions [104]. However, the sites or substrates of the coordination between reaching and grasping are still a matter of debate.

(3) The bimanual coordination, which belongs to the human and primate natural behavior in general. Wiesendanger and co-workers have recently started to investigate this behavior and look for invariances between trajectory and speed of the two hands in a task consisting of pulling a drawer open with one hand and picking up something out of the drawer with the other (fig. 6). On the basis of earlier investigations [105], it was assumed that the site of bimanual coordination would be located in the SMA. However, until now, the neuronal activity in the SMA during the bimanual task has not given strong support to that hypothesis [106].

The review written by Wiesendanger [57] in 1986 and a recent one in 1993 [107] both perfectly reflect the evolution of the interests of the author and illustrate the path he covered in the last 10–15 years: from the role of the SMA in the gating of proprioceptive afferences to the motor cortex, the somatotopical organization of this area as seen by microstimulation, its input-output linkage and its connectivity at the anatomical and physiological level to the function of the SMA in movement initiation and, finally, in the coordination of bimanual behavior in awake monkeys. This evolution closely follows the development of the research trends discussed previously.

From all the questions asked at the end of the 1981 review, very few have yet been answered, and many may even remain without answer for some time, because more important issues have now priority.

Perspective

For this last section, two mottoes have been chosen, *'at the conquest of the space-time'* and *'the future has already started'*.

The technical progresses of the last years, mainly of the last decade, have had an important influence on the concepts which underlay neuroscience research. In particular,

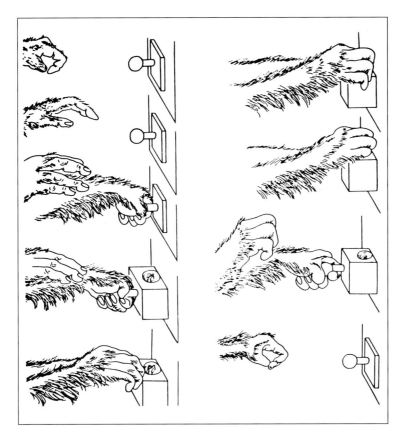

Fig. 6. Bimanual pull-and-grasp synergy. Movement sequence from top to bottom. First, left arm reaching for the knob of the drawer and pulling it. Then, movement of right arm with hand reaching and picking up food in the drawer, followed by the retraction of the hand. (From Wiesendanger [109], with permission.)

powerful computers and software can now simulate complex processes with a precision and spatiotemporal resolution that were previously inconceivable. A simple structure such as the PT is no longer interesting, but this is the ensemble of many structures and their dynamical interactions which is now polarizing the scientific interest.

The first conquest of the space-time is the study and representation of complex and natural movements. The new techniques give now the possibility to measure all the phases of a complex motor behavior, both temporally and spatially [108, 109], to describe natural motor behaviors under all their aspects, and thus to investigate in human subjects and patients the interdependent modifications of the various parts of the body during postural adaptations [Massion, chap. 4] or during locomotion [Dietz, chap. 5]. This experimental approach has the advantage of being totally noninvasive, and can therefore be applied in animals as in human subjects.

The second conquest of the space-time is the recording of the neuronal activity with multiple electrodes in one or several regions of the brain simultaneously. Such an approach, which gives access to networks and their operation, is a promising tool and is likely to yield a better understanding of the systems in general and the motor system in particular. This type of investigation still requires major developments, mainly at the level of the data processing, if some concepts of universal value are to be extracted out of the large amount of data. Though a difficult problem to attack, multicellular recordings are absolutely unavoidable if we are to elucidate the spatiotemporal linkage of the many neuronal populations that participate in various regions of the brain to specific motor tasks [110–112]. This technique, coupled to the detailed measurements of motor behavior described above, will create the possibility to relate neuronal activity to behavior itself, rather than to one restricted parameter of movement.

The third conquest of the space-time is provided by all the techniques of cerebral imaging. Here one can almost tell that science is on its way to overtake fiction. The functional magnetic resonance imaging (fMRI) promises to show the localization of certain processes not only with great precision, but also, in a not too distant future, their modifications in real time. Coupled to electroencephalography and magnetoencephalography, brain imaging should give the possibility to correlate the activity of whole networks with motor behavior in space and time. Positron emission tomography and fMRI have already opened some windows on the cerebral activity in humans during movement execution [113], motor learning [114–116] and motor imagery [117, 118]. At present all these images are static, or taken at various moments of a motor task. The time factor still needs to be added if the controversial issue of hierarchical versus parallel organization is to be solved. The answer to this fundamental question is maybe not too far ahead, and, in contrast to other investigations, it will be given for the human brain – the final subject of all our preoccupations.

The breadth and power of the new methods considered here will inevitably help in answering some of the questions raised by Wiesendanger in his 1981 review, such as the enigma of the motor recuperation and of the substituting pathways. Recent data already suggest that the contingent of corticospinal axons with their origin in the ipsilateral and/or the lateral premotor cortex may play a major role in the reorganization which takes place, for example, after capsular infarcts [119]. Investigations with magnetic transcranial stimulation [Hess et al., chap. 9] already support the role of the ipsilateral pathway in motor recovery [120]. Moreover, these new noninvasive techniques will make explicit the temporal and spatial processes of central reorganization, following either the section of peripheral nerves or after extensive use, discovered in animals for the cortical somatosensory and motor maps [121–123].

All these conquests will stay at the descriptive level if theoretical and technical efforts do not occur in parallel. This is where neuroinformatics and computational neuroscience, with powerful simulations, realistic neuronal networks, and robotics will be absolutely necessary if we are to make sense of the wealth of observations provided by the new techniques discussed here.

Conclusion

Wiesendanger, to whom this chapter is dedicated, has travelled for more than 30 years of the history of the pyramidal tract. On many occasions he has made history himself, together with his collaborators. In 1994, at a strategic historical moment, he leaped into the future, coming back to the past, that is to the study of Man and of patients, where the history of research into pyramidal tract had begun more than a century earlier.

The influence of the following remark made by Sherrington, quoted by Walshe [14] in 1947 and found in several publications of Wiesendanger, has surely not played a minor role in this decision: *'You chose a hard question and one which the bedside is far better place to solve than the laboratory, I think. The pyramidal tract is such a human feature'* [p. 330].

References

1   Magendie FJ: Le ons sur les fonctions et les maladies du système nerveux. Paris, Chez Ebrard, 1839, vol 1, p 282.
2   Lassek AM: The PT. Its Status in Medicine. Springfield, Thomas, 1954.
3   Hepp-Reymond MC: Functional organization of motor cortex and its participation in voluntary movement; in Comparative Primate Biology, vol 4: Neurosciences. New York, Liss, 1988, pp 501–624.
4   Pourfour du Petit F: Lettre d'un médecin des hôpitaux du Roi à un autre médecin de ses amis. Namur, 1710.
5   Gall FJ, Spurzheim JC: Anatomie et physiologie du système nerveux en général, et du cerveau en particulier. Paris, Schoell et al, 1810–1819.
6   Türck L: Über sekundäre Erkrankungen einzelner Rückenmarkstränge und ihrer Fortsetzung zum Gehirne. Z Kaiserl Königl Ges Ärzte Wien 1851;8:511–534.
7   Cruveilhier J: The Anatomy of the Human Body. New York, Harper Bros, 1853.
8   Fritsch G, Hitzig E: Über die elektrische Erregbarkeit des Grosshirns. Arch Anat Physiol Wiss Med (Leipzig) 1870;37:300–332.
9   Ferrier D: Experimental researches in cerebral physiology and pathology. West Riding Lunatic Asylum Med Rep 1873;3:1–50.
10 Broca PP: Remarques sur le siège de la faculté du langage articulé, suivie d'une observation d'aphémie (Perte de la parole). Bull Soc Anat Paris 1861;36:330–357.
11 Sherrington CS: On nerve-tracts degeneration secondarily to lesions of the cortex cerebri. J Neurophysiol (Lond) 1889;10:429–432.
12 Betz VA: Anatomischer Nachweis zweier Gehirncentra. Centralbl Med Wiss 1874;12:578–580, 595–599.
13 Walshe FMR: The giant cells of Betz, the motor cortex and the PT: A critical review. Brain 1942;65:409–462.
14 Walshe FMR: On the role of the pyramidal system in willed movements. Brain 1947;70:329–354.
15 Wiesendanger M: The PT. Recent investigations on its morphology and function; in Ergebnisse der Physiologie, Biologischen Chemie und experimentellen Pharmakologie. Berlin, Springer, 1969, pp 73–136.
16 Phillips CG, Porter R: The pyramidal projection to motoneurons of some muscle groups of the baboon's forelimb. Prog Brain Res 1964;12:222–242.
17 Buser P, Ascher P: Mise en jeu réflexe du système pyramidal chez le chat. Arch Ital Biol 1960;98:123–164.
18 Brooks VB: Some factors governing sensory convergence in the cat's motor cortex; in Studies in Physiology. Berlin, Springer, 1965, p 13.
19 Eccles JC: Cerebral synaptic mechanism; in Eccles JC (ed): Brain and Conscious Experience. Berlin, Springer, 1966.
20 Evarts EV: Pyramidal tract activity associated with a conditioned hand movement in the monkey. J Neurophysiol 1966;29:1011–1027.
21 Evarts EV: Relation of pyramidal tract activity to force exerted during voluntary movements. J Neurophysiol 1968;31:14–27.
22 Evarts EV: Representation of movements and muscles by pyramidal tract neurons of the precentral motor cortex; in Yahr MD, Purpura DP (eds): Neurophysiological Basis of Normal and Abnormal Motor Activities. New York, Raven Press, 1967, pp 215–251.
23 Jackson JH: On the comparative study of diseases of the nervous system. Br Med J 1889;ii:355–362. Reprinted 1932; in Selected Writings of John Hughlings Jackson 1932;2:939–410.
24 Philips CG: Changing concepts of the precentral motor area; in Eccles J (ed): Brain and Conscious Experience. Berlin, Springer, 1966, pp 389–421.
25 Lawrence DG, Kuypers HGJM: The functional organization of the motor system in the monkey. I. The effects of bilateral pyramidal lesions. Brain 1968;91:1–14.
26 Hepp-Reymond MC, Wiesendanger M: Unilateral pyramidotomy in monkeys: Effect on force and speed of a contioned rapid precision grip in monkeys. Brain Res 1972;36:117–131.
27 Chapman CE, Wiesendanger M: Recovery of function following unilateral lesions of the bulbar pyramid in the monkey. Electroencephalogr Clin Neurophysiol 1982;53:374–387.
28 Tower SS: Pyramidal lesions in the monkey. Brain 1940;63:36–90.
29 Wiesendanger M: The pyramidal tract. Its structure and function; in Towe AL, Luschei ES (eds): Handbook of Behavioral Neurobiology. New York, Plenum Press, 1981, vol 5, pp 401–491.
30 Hepp-Reymond MC, Trouche E, Wiesendanger M: Effects of unilateral und bilateral pyramidotomy on a conditioned rapid precision grip in monkeys. Exp Brain Res 1974;21:519–527.
31 Bruckmoser P, Hepp-Reymond MC, Wiesendanger M: Cortical influence on single neurons of the lateral reticular nucleus of the cat. Exp Neurol 1970;26:239–252.

32   Wiesendanger M, Rüegg DG, Wiesendanger R: The corticopontine system in primates: Anatomical and physiological considerations; in Massion J, Sasaki K (eds): Cerebro-Cerebellar Interactions. Amsterdam, Elsevier, 1979, pp 45–65.

33   Keizer K, Kuypers HGJM: Distribution of corticospinal neurons with collaterals to the lower brain stem reticular formation; in monkey (*Macaca fascicularis*). Exp Brain Res 1989;74:311–318.

34   Asanuma H: Recent developments in the study of the columnar arrangement of neurons within the motor cortex. Physiol Rev 1975;55:143–156.

35   Wiesendanger M: Input from muscle and cutaneous nerves of the hand and forearm to neurons of the precentral gyrus of baboon and monkeys. J Physiol (Lond) 1973;228:203–219.

36   Phillips CG, Porter R: Corticospinal Neurones. London, Academic Press, 1977.

37   Philips CG: Motor apparatus of the baboon's hand. Proc R Soc Lond [B] 1969;173:141–174.

38   Conrad B, Matsunami K, Meyer-Lohmann J, Wiesendanger M, Brooks VB: Cortical load compensation during voluntary elbow movements. Brain Res 1974;71:507–514.

39   Evarts EV: Motor cortex reflexes associated with learned movement. Science 1973;179:501–503.

40   Evarts EV, Tanji J: Gating of motor cortex reflexes by prior instruction. Brain Res 1974;71:479–94.

41   Wiesendanger M, Rüegg DG, Lucier GE: Why transcortical reflexes? Can J Neurol Sci 1975;2:295–301.

42   Wiesendanger M: Comments on the problem of transcortical reflexes. J Physiol (Paris) 1978;74:325–330.

43   Cheney PD, Fetz EE: Corticomotoneuronal cells contribute to long-latency stretch reflex in the rhesus monkey. J Physiol (Lond) 1984;349:249–272.

44   Shinoda Y, Zarzecki P, Asanuma H: Spinal branching of PT neurons in the monkey. Exp Brain Res 1979;34: 59–72.

45   Shinoda Y, Yokota J, Fumati T: Divergent projection of individual corticospinal axons to motoneurons of multiple muscles in the monkey. Neurosci Lett 1981;23:7–12.

46   Fetz EE, Cheney PD: Post-spike facilitation of forelimb muscle activity by primate corticomotoneuronal cells. J Neurophysiol 1980;44:751–772.

47   Smith AM, Hepp-Reymond MC, Wyss UR: Relation of activity in precentral cortical neurons to force and rate of force change during isometric contractions of finger muscles. Exp Brain Res 1975;23:315–332.

48   Hepp-Reymond MC, Wyss UR, Anner R: Neuronal coding of static force in the primate motor cortex. J Physiol (Paris) 1978;74:287–291.

49   Thach WT: Correlation of neural discharge with pattern and force of muscular activity, joint position and direction of intended next movement in motor cortex and cerebellum. J Neurophysiol 1978;41:654–676.

50   Evarts EV, Fromm C: The PTN summing point in a closed-loop control system in the monkey. Prog Clin Neurophysiol 1978;4:56–69.

51   Evarts EV: Activity of motor cortex (MI) neurons during voluntary movements in the monkey; in Brooks VB (ed): Handbook of Physiology. The Nervous System. Bethesda, American Physiological Society, 1981, part 2, pp 1083–1120.

52   Wiesendanger M: Organization of secondary motor areas of cerebral cortex; in Brooks VB (ed): Handbook of Physiology. The Nervous System. Bethesda, American Physiological Society, 1981, part 2, pp 1121–1147.

53   Wiesendanger M, Séguin JJ, Künzle H: The supplementary motor area – a control system for posture? in Stein RB, Pearson KG, Smith RS, Redford JB (eds): Control of Posture and Locomotion. New York, Plenum Press, 1973, pp 331–346.

54   Tanji J, Taniguchi K: Does the supplementary motor area play a part in modifying motor cortex reflexes? J Physiol 1978;74:317–318.

55   Evarts EV, Shinoda Y, Wise SP: Neurophysiological Approaches to Higher Brain Functions. New York, Wiley, 1984.

56   Wise SP: Higher Brain Functions. New York, Wiley, 1987.

57   Wiesendanger M: Recent developments in studies of the supplementary motor area in primates. Rev Physiol Biochem Pharmacol 1986;193:1–59.

58   Roland PE, Larsen B, Lassen NA, Skinhoj E: Supplementary motor area and other cortical areas in organization of voluntary movements in man. J Neurophysiol 1980;43:118–136.

59   Porter R, Lemon R: Corticospinal function and voluntary movement; in Monographs of the Physiological Society. Oxford Science Publications. Oxford, Clarendon Press, 1993, vol 45.

60   Dum RP, Strick PL: The origin of corticospinal projections from the premotor areas in the frontal lobe. J Neurosci 1991;11:667–689.

61   Murphy JT, Kwan HC, MacKay WA, Wong YC: Spatial organization of precentral cortex in awake primates. III. Input-output coupling. J Neurophysiol 1978;41:1132–1139.

62   Sessle BJ, Wiesendanger M: Structural and functional definition of the motor cortex in the monkey (*Macaca fascicularis*). J Physiol (Lond) 1982;323:245–265.

63   Lemon RN, Hanby JA, Porter R: Relationship between the activity of precentral neurones during active and passive movements in conscious monkeys. Proc R Soc Lond [B] 1976;194:341–373.

64   Strick PL, Preston JB: Sorting of somatosensory afferent information in primate motor cortex. Brain Res 1978; 156:364–368.

65   Wiesendanger M: The motor cortical areas and the problem of hierarchies; in Jeannerod M (ed): Attention and Performance. XIII. Motor Representation and Control. Hillsdale, Erlbaum Associates, 1990, pp 59–75.

66   Schell GR, Strick PL: The origin of thalamic inputs to the arcuate premotor and supplementary motor areas. J Neurosci 1984;4:539–560.

67   Wiesendanger R, Wiesendanger M: The thalamic connections with medial area 6 (supplementary motor cortex) in the monkey. Exp Brain Res 1985;56:91–104.
68   Wiesendanger R, Wiesendanger M: Cerebello-cortical linkage in the monkey as revealed by transcellular labelling with the lectin wheat germ agglutinin conjugated to the marker horseradish peroxidase. Exp Brain Res 1985; 56:105–117.
69   Dum RP, Strick PL: Premotor areas: Nodal points for efferent system involved in central control of movement; in Humphrey DR, Freund JH (eds): Motor Control: Concepts and Issues. Chichester, Wiley, 1991, pp 383–398.
70   Tanji J: The supplementary motor area in the cerebral cortex. Neurosci Res 1994;19:251–268.
71   Passingham RE: Two cortical systems for directing movement; in Motor Areas of the Cerebral Cortex. Chichester, Wiley, 1987, pp 151–164.
72   Halsband U, Freund HJ: Premotor cortex and conditional motor learning in man. Brain 1990;113:207–222.
73   Anner-Baratti R, Allum JHJ, Hepp-Reymond MC: Neural correlates of isometric force in the 'motor' thalamus. Exp Brain Res 1986;63:567–580.
74   Wannier TMJ, Maier MA, Hepp-Reymond MC: Contrasting properties of monkey somatosensory and motor cortex neurons activated during the control of force in precision grip. J Physiol 1991;65:572–589.
75   Hepp-Reymond MC, Hüsler EJ, Maier MA, Qi HX: Force-related neuronal activity in two regions of the primate ventral premotor cortex. Can J Physiol Pharmacol 1994;72:571–579.
76   Alexander GE, Crutcher MD: Preparation for movement: Neural representations of intended direction in three motor areas of the monkey. J Neurophysiol 1990;64:133–150.
77   Riehle A, Requin J: Monkey primary motor and premotor cortex: Single-cell activity related to prior information about direction and extent of an intended movement. J Neurophysiol 1989;61:534–549.
78   Riehle A, MacKay WA, Requin J: Are extent and force independent movement parameters? Preparation- and movement-related neuronal activity in the monkey cortex. Exp Brain Res 1994;99:56–74.
79   Kalaska JF: What parameters of reaching are encoded by discharges of cortical cells? in Humphrey DR, Freund JH (eds): Motor Control: Concepts and Issues. Chichester, Wiley, 1991, pp 307–330.
80   Chen DF, Hyland B, Maier V, Palmeri A, Wiesendanger M: Comparison of neuronal activity in the supplementary motor area and in the primary motor cortex in monkey. Somatosens Mot Res 1991;8:27–44.
81   Fu QG, Suarez JI, Ebner TJ: Neuronal specification of direction and distance during reaching movements in the superior precentral premotor area and primary motor cortex of monkeys. J Neurophysiol 1993;70:2097–2116.
82   Humphrey DR, Tanji J: What features of voluntary motor control are encoded in the neuronal discharge of different cortical motor areas? in Humphrey DR, Freund JH (eds): Motor Control: Concepts and Issues. Chichester, Wiley, 1991, pp 413–443.
83   Seal J, Riehle A, Requin J: A critical re-examination of the concept of function within the neocortex of the monkey. Hum Mov Sci 1992;11:47–58.
84   Georgopoulos AP, Kalaska JF, Caminiti R, Massey JT: On the relations between the direction of two-dimensional arm movements and cell discharge in primate motor cortex. J Neurosci 1982;2:1527–1537.
85   Georgopoulos AP, Schwartz AB, Kettner RE: Neuronal population coding of movement direction. Science 1986;233:1416–1419.
86   Caminiti R, Johnson BP, Galli C, Ferraina S, Burnod Y: Making arm movements within different parts of space: The premotor and motor cortical representation of a coordinate system for reaching to visual targets. J Neurosci 1991;11:1182–1197.
87   Kalaska JF, Crammond DJ: Cerebral cortical mechanisms for reaching movements. Science 1992;255:1517–1523.
88   Georgopoulos AP: New concepts in generation of movement. Neuron 1994;13:257–268.
89   Scott SH, Kalaska JF: Changes in motor cortex activity during reaching movements with similar hand paths but different arm postures. J Neurophysiol 1995;73:2563–2567.
90   Lacquaniti F, Guignon E, Bianchi L, Ferraina S, Caminiti R: Representing spatial information for limb movement: Role of area 5 in the monkey. Cereb Cortex 1995;5:391–409.
91   Wise SP: The primate premotor cortex: Past, present and preparatory. Annu Rev Neurosci 1985;8:1–19.
92   Mushiake H, Inase M, Tanji J: Neural activity in the primate premotor supplementary and precentral motor cortex during visually guided and internally determined sequential movements. J Neurophysiol 1991;66:705–718.
93   Tanji J, Kurata K: Changing concepts of motor areas of the cerebral cortex. Brain Dev 1989;11:374–377.
94   Crammond DJ, Kalaska JF: Modulation of preparatory neuronal activity in dorsal premotor cortex due to stimulus-response compatibility. J Neurophysiol 1994;71:1281–1284.
95   di Pellegrino G, Wise SP: Visuospatial versus visuomotor activity in the premotor and prefrontal cortex of a primate. J Neurosci 1993;13:1227–1243.
96   Boussaoud D, Wise SP: Primate frontal cortex: Neuronal activity following attentional versus intentional cues. Exp Brain Res 1993;95:15–27.
97   Qi HX, Hüsler EJ, Alig I, Hepp-Reymond MC: Simple and complex relations of motor cortical activity to grip force in the alert monkey. Soc Neurosci Abstr 1994;20:981.
98   Tanji J, Shima K: Role for supplementary motor area cells in planning several movements ahead. Nature 1994; 371:413–416.
99   Lemon RN, Bennett KM, Werner W: The cortico-motor substrate for skilled movements of the primate hand; in Requin J, Stelmach GE (eds): Tutorials in Motor Neuroscience. Dordrecht, Kluwer Academic Publishers, 1991, pp 477–495.

100 Johansson RS: How is grasping modified by somatosensory input? in Humphrey DR, Freund JH (eds): Motor Control: Concepts and Issues. Chichester, Wiley, 1991, pp 331–356.

101 Picard N, Smith AM: Primary motor cortical activity related to the weight and texture of grasped objects in the monkey. J Neurophysiol 1992;68:1867–1881.

102 Smith AM: Some shear facts and pure friction related to roughness discrimination and the cutaneous control of grasping. Can J Physiol Pharmacol 1994;72:583–590.

103 Jeannerod M: The formation of finger grip during prehension. A cortically mediated visuomotor pattern. Behav Brain Res 1986;19:99–116.

104 Sakata H: Parietal control of hand action. Curr Opin Neurobiol 1994;4:847–856.

105 Brinkman J: Supplementary motor area of the monkey's cerebral cortex: Short- and long-term deficits after unilateral ablation and the effects of subsequent callosal section. J Neurosci 1984;4:918–929.

106 Wiesendanger M, Rouiller EM, Kazennikov O, Perrig S: Is the supplementary motor area a bilaterally organized system? in Lüders HO (ed): Advances in Neurology, vol 70: Supplementary Sensorimotor Area. Philadelphia, Lippincott-Raven, 1996, pp 85–93.

107 Wiesendanger M: The riddle of supplementary area function; in Mano N, Hamada I, DeLong MR (eds): Role of the Cerebellum and Basal Ganglia in Voluntary Movement. Amsterdam, Elsevier, 1993, pp 253–266.

108 Jeannerod M, Paulignan Y, Mackenzie C, Marteniuk RM: Parallel visuomotor processing in human prehension movements; in Caminiti R, Johnson PB, Burnod Y (eds): Control of Arm Movement in Space. Berlin, Springer, 1992, pp 27–44.

109 Wiesendanger M, Corboz M, Hyland B, Palmeri A, Maier V, Wicki U, Rouiller E: Bimanual synergies in primates; in Caminiti R, Johnson PB, Burnod Y (eds): Control of Arm Movement in Space. Berlin, Springer, 1992, pp 45–64.

110 Aertsen AM, Gerstein GL, Habib MK, Palm G: Dynamics of neuronal firing correlation: Modulation of 'effective connectivity'. J Neurophysiol 1989;61:900–917.

111 Riehle A, Seal J, Requin J, Grün S, Aertsen A: Multi-electrode recording of neuronal activity in the motor cortex: Evidence for changes in the functional coupling between neurons; in Herrmann HJ, Wolf DE, Pöppel E (eds): Supercomputing in Brain Research: from Tomography to Neural Networks. Singapore, World Scientific, 1995, pp 281–288.

112 Seidemann E, Meilijson I, Abeles M, Bergman H, Vaadia E: Simultaneously recorded single units in the frontal cortex go through sequences of discrete and stable states in monkeys performing a delayed localization task. J Neurosci 1996;16:752–768.

113 Colebatch JG, Deiber MP, Passingham RE, Friston KJ, Frackowiak RSJ: Regional cerebral blood flow during voluntary arm and hand movements in human subjects. J Neurophysiol 1991;65:1392–1401.

114 Grafton ST, Mazziotta JC, Presty S, Friston KJ, Frackowiak SJ, Phelps ME: Functional anatomy of human procedural learning determined with regional cerebral blood flow and PET. J Neurosci 1992;12:2542–2548.

115 Seitz RJ, Roland PE: Learning of sequential finger movements in man: A combined kinematic and positron emission tomography study. Eur J Neurosci 1992;4:154–165.

116 Karni A, Meyer G, Jezzard P, Adams MM, Turner R, Ungerleider LG: Functional MRI evidence for adult motor cortex plasticity during motor skill learning. Nature 1995;377:155–158.

117 Décéty J, Perani D, Jeannerod M, Betttinardi V, Tadary B, Woods R, Mazziotta JC, Fazio F: Mapping motor representations with positron emission tomography. Nature 1994;371:600–602.

118 Stephan KM, Fink GR, Passingham RE, Silbersweig D, Ceballos-Baumann AO, Frith CD, Frackowiak RSJ: Functional anatomy of the mental representation of upper extremity movements in healthy subjects. J Neurophysiol 1995;73:373–386.

119 Chollet F, DiPiero V, Wise RJ, Brooks DJ, Dolan RJ, Frackowiak RS: The functional anatomy of motor recovery after stroke in humans: A study with positron emission tomography. Ann Neurol 1991;29:63–71.

120 Fries W, Danek A, Scheidtmann K, Hamburger C: Motor recovery following capsular stroke. Brain 1993;116: 369–382.

121 Merzenich MM: Dynamic neocortical processes and the origins of higher brain functions; in Changeux JP, Konishi M (eds): The Neural and Molecular Bases of Learning. Chichester, Wiley, 1987, pp 337–358.

122 Sanes JN, Donoghue JP: Organization and adaptability of muscle representations in primary motor cortex; in Caminiti R, Johnson PB, Burnod Y (eds): Control of Arm Movement in Space. Berlin, Springer, 1992, pp 103–127.

123 Nudo RJ, Milliken GW, Jenkins WM, Merzenich MM: Use-dependent alterations of movement representations in primary motor cortex of adult squirrel monkeys. J Neurophysiol 1996;16:785–807.

Dr. Marie-Claude Hepp-Reymond, Brain Research Institute, University of Zürich,
August-Forel-Strasse 1, CH–8029 Zürich (Switzerland)

Hepp-Reymond M-C, Marini G (eds): Perspectives of Motor Behavior and Its Neural Basis.
Basel, Karger, 1997, pp 19–32

....

Grasping Objects: The Hand as a Pattern Recognition Device

Marc Jeannerod

Vision et Motricité, INSERM U94, Bron, France

Human motor skills culminate in the ability to generate highly coordinated action patterns with multiple-joint musculoskeletal systems like the vocal tract or the hand. For this reason, hand movements have been the focus of interest of many researchers since the origins of neuroscience. In his treatise on the hand, Charles Bell [1] compared hand movements with eye movements, which both have the same function of bringing objects on the most sensitive part of the sensory surface for the purpose of analysis and recognition. The hand is at the interface between visual and tactile analysis. Although its movements toward objects are dictated, for the most part, by vision, it becomes a tactile organ as soon as contact is made. Berkeley [2] in his famous treatise on 'A new theory of vision', emphasized the fact that objects can only be known by touch, which he considered as the ultimate means of exploration and knowledge of the world. Vision is subject to illusions, which arise from the distance-size problem (size must be extracted from apparent distance) or the three-dimensional (3-D) reconstruction problem (the visual third dimension is extracted from a two-dimensional map using indirect cues from perspective). Touch, and particularly active touch, is not subject to these constraints, as it involves direct assessment of size and volume. In addition, touch is critical for perceiving object properties like hardness, compliance, texture, temperature, weight, etc., which can hardly be accessed by sight alone.

In this paper, the emphasis will be on movements of the hand in the context of visually-directed grasping. Grasping thus pertains to the broad function of object recognition: not only is it the precondition for handling and manipulation, during which signals arising from sight and touch are coprocessed. It also reflects visuomotor transformation, a process by which the visual attributes of an object are mapped into motor commands.

Description of Grip Patterns

The pattern of finger movements and postures during the action of grasping aims at achieving a stable grasp of the object, as a prerequisite for handling objects. By using this criterion of stability, Napier [3] considered that human prehensile movements can be described along only two main motor patterns. '*If*', Napier stated, '*prehensile activities are to be regarded as the application of a system of forces in a given direction then the nature of prehensile activity can be resolved into two concepts – that of precision and that of power'* [p. 906]. The precision and the power grip patterns can be used alternatively or in combination for almost every object. In other words, the pattern of the grip is not determined (solely) by the shape or the size of the object (e.g., a rod can be held with a precision grip, as in writing, or a power grip, as in hammering); it is the intended activity that is the main determinant of the type of grip for each given action.

The two grips differ anatomically by both the posture of the thumb and the posture of the fingers. Precision grip is mostly characterized by opposition of the thumb to one or more of the other fingers. Opposition means that the thumb is abducted and rotated at the metacarpophalangeal and at the carpometacarpal joints, so that its pulpar surface is diametrically opposed to the pulpar surface of the other fingers. In power grip, the fingers are flexed to form a clamp against the palm, the thumb is adducted at the two joints, and there is no opposition between the thumb and the other fingers. The two types of grip have clearly different degrees of involvement in manipulative actions, only the precision handling allows movements of the object relative to the hand and movements of the object within the hand, because of opposition of the thumb to the other fingers [4].

Precision grip with true opposition of the pulpar surfaces of the thumb and the other fingers is thus considered as the top attribute of dextrous hands. The problem of whether this attribute is specific to the human hand or not, is a matter of discussion. The human hand is the only one to combine the two major attributes that result in dexterity: an opposable thumb and independent fingers. Accordingly, not only can the thumb oppose all the other fingers separately, but also all the available degrees of freedom of the hand can be used in performing the grip, according to the object configuration, or to the requirements of the task. The Heffner and Masterton scale for ranking digital dexterity [5], based on anatomy of the hand, includes only man in the topmost category [see also 6]. Recent work based on fossil anatomical evidence, however, indicates that this category should be extended to remote predecessors of modern humans (e.g., *Paranthropus robustus*, 1.8 million years), which are credited of dextrous tool use behavior [7]. The relative ratio of index finger and thumb length, as well as the position of the articulation of the thumb, have changed from a chimpanzee-like hand in *Australopithecus afarensis* (4 million years) to a modern human-like arrangement in *Homo erectus* (1.5 million years). It should not be concluded from this difference that the other primates are not capable of opposition: they can abduct their thumb and rotate it in front of their other fingers, but the shortness of the thumb in several species prevents contact between the pulpar surfaces [8]. In addition, the classification based on anatomy of the hand is probably underinclusive, and should be counterbalanced by a classification based on behavioral observation with emphasis on the capability for independent finger movements and for the use of tools. Tool use behavior is well known in apes like chimpanzee and orang-utan, [e.g. 9].

Christel [10, 11], in describing the areas of the hand which come in contact with each other during grasping tasks, has made an extensive study of prehensile hands in a variety of primates. Many species are capable of opposing the thumb with the pulpar surface of the index and the side of the third finger. This is the most frequent type of precision grip in chimpanzees, humans, gorillas and orang-utan, in descending order. In addition, side opposition between the pulp of the thumb and the side of the middle or the terminal phalanx of the index finger, or between the side of the thumb and the side of the middle phalanx, is also commonly observed, especially in bonobos and orang-utans (fig. 1). By contrast, according to Christel, the opposition (pulpar or otherwise) of the thumb with the fourth and the fifth fingers is never observed in any of these animals.

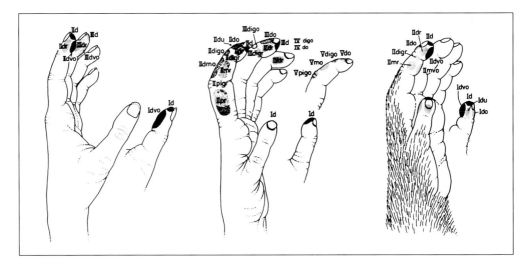

Fig. 1. Areas of contact between fingers during precision grip. Areas of contact have been plotted on a human hand (left), a generalized hand of 6 hominoid species (middle) and a generalized hand of 3 cercopithecid species (right). In the hominoid hand, note the importance of contacts between the tip of the thumb and the lateral aspect of the second finger. Courtesy of Christel [11].

Animals like rhesus monkeys or baboons, or even new-world monkeys like cebus monkeys, are thus capable of accurate precision grips [see 12 for review]. Other still more primitive animals use whole hand prehension with a nonopposable thumb, a good example of which is given by behavioral observation of squirrel monkeys. In this animal, objects are reached with all the fingers in a slightly curved and convergent position; in the later stage of the reach, the fingers diverge and straighten, closing in a scooping motion at contact with the object; the fingers frequently close to the palm with the distal and medial phalanges parallel to the palm, rather than curled around the objects as human fingers do [13]. Interestingly, this description of a primitive prehensile behavior can be applied almost without change to pathological prehension in higher primates following motor cortical lesions [14–16]. This observation predicts that the various types of grasps displayed by infra-human species relate to different degrees of cortical control of the hand muscles. This was indeed nicely demonstrated in a recent paper by Bortoff and Strick [17]. They found that the corticospinal terminations on the motoneurons controlling the finger muscles markedly differed in two of the above mentioned monkey species with different grasping capabilities: dense terminations were observed in the cebus, while they were practically absent in squirrel monkeys. This reminds us that *'the increasing versatility of hand function as we ascend the primate scale has been conferred by a progressive enlargement of cerebral cortex and cerebellum and a corresponding enrichment of their intrinsic and extrinsic synaptic connectivity'* [18, p. 6].

The Selection of Object Attributes Relevant to Grasping

This section deals with the selection of the object attributes that must be taken into account for designing the appropriate final configuration of the hand. This mode of processing visual and haptic information for the purpose of interacting with objects differs from that used for comparing, naming, or memorizing objects. The term of 'pragmatic' processing (as opposed to 'semantic' processing) has been used to highlight its specificity [see 19].

An essential aspect of pragmatic processing is visuomotor transformation. To ensure a stable grasp, the hand must rotate and bring the grip at the proper orientation, grip size must relate to the size of the object, intervening fingers must be selected according to its 3-D properties, etc., so that the force vectors applied by the fingers on the object should be in exactly opposite directions. In the case of handling a cylindrical object like a glass, for example, the fingers will have to be placed at the two ends of the same diameter in order to achieve a stable grasp. This selection implies the existence of higher order visuomotor mechanisms for extracting from the object the parameters that are both constituent of its shape and relevant to the generation of the appropriate motor commands. Among those parameters are area, gravicenter, length of vectors, orientation of surfaces, etc. Recent neurophysiological data in monkey may account for this possibility. Neurons located in parietal area 7 have been shown to detect the size, length and orientation of objects. They may also be specifically activated by broad categories, such as cylindrical vs. spherical shapes [20]. In addition, other neurons in a nearby area have been shown to be activated prior to reaching movements directed at objects of a given orientation or shape [21]. These neurons, located in a region which is directly connected to premotor cortex, may therefore represent the neural mechanism for transferring the visually perceived orientation into a motor code. These data clearly suggest that there are at least two mechanisms for detecting object shape. The mechanisms located in the parietal cortex would therefore represent the neural substrate for pragmatic processing, i.e., for processing those aspects of shape which are relevant to interaction with objects.

For the sake of reducing the many degrees of freedom involved in the complex motor pattern of grasping, a coordinated control program, extending that used in computational models, has been proposed. This approach [22–25] assumes the existence of preorganized motor 'schemas' which determine the interactions between the hand and the environment. For the purpose of prehension, schemas like 'preshape', 'enclose', 'orient', etc. are postulated. These schemas are carried out by specific grasping units (the 'virtual fingers'). In a precision grip with pad opposition, for example, the virtual fingers are the thumb (VF1), the finger(s) that oppose the thumb (VF2), and the unused finger(s) (VF3). In grasping a small object, VF2 will be composed of the index finger only. In whole hand prehension with palm opposition, VF1 will be the palm and VF2 will (usually) include the four fingers other than the thumb. The role of vision in activating the proper schemas and specifying the composition of the virtual fingers, is to determine the relative positions of the hand and the object to be grasped, so that the forces during the lift of the object can be applied in exactly opposite directions. This requires defining an 'opposition space' corresponding to the grasp axis embedded in the object. Then, the hand will be transported (the 'approach' schema) and the wrist will rotate it (the 'rotate' schema) in order to approximate the correct position. The sections below will describe two of these behavioral patterns, related to matching object size and orientation, respectively.

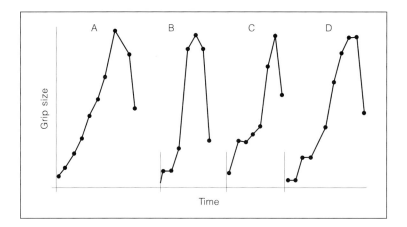

Fig. 2. Pattern of grip formation in one macaque monkey. The distance between the tip of the index finger and the tip of the thumb (grip size) has been plotted during four grasping movements (**A–D**). The animal was forming a precision grip for grasping small pieces of food. The rightmost point on each movement was plotted when either finger came in contact with the food. Note progressive opening of grip and sharp closure before contact with the object. Data from successive frames on a film taken at 25 frames per second. Courtesy of S. Faugier-Grimaud.

Matching Object Size

The type of grip that is formed by the hand in contact with the object represents the end result of a motor sequence which starts well ahead of the action of grasping itself. The fingers preshape according to object size during transportation of the hand at the object location.

Preshaping first involves a progressive opening of the grip with straightening of the fingers, followed by a closure of the grip until it matches object size. The point in time where grip size is the largest (maximum grip size) is a clearly identifiable landmark which occurs within about 60–70% of the duration of the reach, that is, well before the fingers come in contact with the object [26–30]. This motor pattern is not unique to man: observations based on films during prehension in one rhesus monkey have revealed a closely similar opening of the grip followed by closure before contact with the object (fig. 2).

One possible explanation for this biphasic opening-closure pattern of grip formation relates to the thumb-index finger geometry. Because the index finger is longer than the thumb, the finger grip has to open wider than required by object size, in order for the index finger to turn around the object and to achieve the proper orientation of the grip. Indeed, the movement of the index contributes the most to grip formation, whereas the position of the thumb with respect to the wrist tends to remain invariant (within limits [31]). The extra-opening of the grip during preshaping might also represent a safety margin for compensating the effects of the variability of the reach. Indeed, maximum grip size tends to become larger than required by object size in a number of conditions where the variability of the reach is likely to be increased (e.g., lack of visual control, movements directed at targets in the peripheral visual field, etc.). This point will be discussed below.

The pattern of grip formation, however, should not be reduced to a biomechanical problem. Preshaping indeed reflects a high-order visual mechanism for processing object attributes: this is demonstrated by the fact that the amplitude of grip aperture during grip

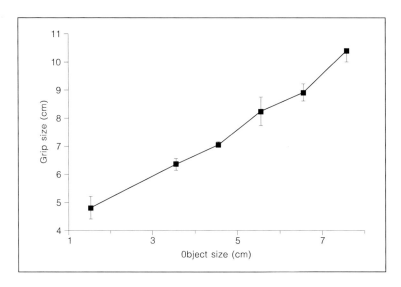

Fig. 3. Change in maximum grip size as a function of object size. Distance between the tip of the index and the tip of the thumb was plotted at the time of maximum grip aperture in one normal subject during grasping movements directed at objects of different sizes. The rate of aperture (measured as the mean increase in grip aperture for 1 cm increase in object size) was 0.95 cm; i.e., close to the 0.77 cm value noted by Marteniuk et al. [32], in a population of normal subjects.

formation covaries with object size [27–29]. Marteniuk et al. [32] found that for an increase of 1 cm in object size, the maximum grip size increases by 0.77 cm (fig. 3). This is an important finding, as the rate of grip aperture during preshape can be used as an index of the functioning of the visual system responsible for pragmatic processing and ultimately for visuomotor transformation [e.g., 33].

These results raise the problem of the accuracy of visuomotor transformation for hand and finger movements during grasping. Accuracy, a currently used parameter for assessing motor performance, can easily be quantified in situations like aiming or reaching. This is not the case in natural prehensive movements, where the terminal error in finger position during the grasp is likely to integrate the errors intervening at the level of the other segments of the arm. It is thus necessary, in order to determine the accuracy of the grip component in itself, to use experimental situations where the grip component would be disconnected from, and therefore unperturbed by the other components of prehension.

Jeannerod and Decety [34] undertook such an experiment where they examined the accuracy of finger movements in matching the size of visually presented objects. Feedback cues arising from execution of the movement were excluded as much as possible, by preventing both vision of the performing hand and contact of that hand with the target objects. Thus, subjects had to match the size of their finger grip to the size of objects presented through a mirror precluding vision of their hand. The distance between the tip of the index finger and the tip of the thumb was measured. The results showed that, in spite of a general trend toward overestimation, the mean grip size correlated positively and linearly with target size with high correlation coefficients.

It is interesting to compare the present results with those obtained in psychophysical experiments testing the subjective scaling of visual length or size. It has been proposed that perceived length of a line should be proportional to its physical length, and should not follow a logarithmic function as it is the case in the perception of other physical dimensions. This contention revealed true. The subjective scaling of area, however, has been found by several authors to be related to physical size by a power function with an exponent of 0.7–0.8 [35, 36]. The discrepancy between reports on subjective scaling of length and area might relate to the type of instructions given to the subjects. Teghtsoonian [37] showed that, if subjects were required to estimate the 'objective area' of circles (How large are the circles?), their judgements followed a linear relation to physical size, as it was found for the lines. In contrast, if the task was to estimate the 'apparent size' of the same circles (How large they look to you?), then their judgements followed a power function (exponent 0.76) with respect to physical size. The Jeannerod and Decety [34] results, showing that visuomotor estimation of size is linearly related to target size, therefore suggest that visuomotor transformation actually 'reads' objective size rather than apparent size.

Matching Object Orientation

Consider an elongated object which can be grasped only by opposing the index and thumb pads along its long side. If this object rests horizontally on a table surface and parallel to the subject midline, it can easily be grasped with the right hand in its natural, semipronated, position. However, if the object is rotated clockwise to a position well beyond being parallel to the frontal plane, in order for it to be grasped, the finger opposition space must be realigned to match the afforded graspable surface. This realignment is accomplished through pronation of the forearm as well as by rotation at the glenohumeral joint (which involves both internal rotation and abduction). When full rotation is required the opposition space is realigned such that the thumb and index finger change their relative positions to the midline, i.e., the thumb is now right and the index finger left.

An experiment was performed where the same object was presented at different orientations [38]. For the object angles of 70, 80 and 90°, almost all the grasps were executed without realignment of the opposition space. As the angle increased to 100°, a mixed manner of grasping developed, approximately half of the trials now contained a forearm rotation. With the larger angles of 110 and 120°, the inconsistency disappeared as the subjects systematically added a pronation to the transport phase. Out of 240 object grasps performed by the subjects for these two orientations, only three showed no pronation (fig. 4). This result reveals that the visuomotor system is able to recognize at which orientation angle a pronation is required to grasp the object. At certain critical angles a visuomotor decision is made to rotate the forearm. This categorical visuomotor behavior provides support for the above concept of schemas proposed by Arbib [22, 24]. Schemas may, in addition, be embedded into broader visuomotor strategies such as optimizing the smoothness of the movement or minimizing discomfort by avoiding extreme joint angles, as was proposed recently [39, 40].

An additional argument for the existence of this 'pragmatic' visual processing is that the pattern of grip formation is correctly achieved, i.e., the size of the maximum grip aperture correlates with the size of the object and the proper orientation is selected, in situations where the hand remains invisible to the subject [27]. Visual feedback signals thus seem of little importance during the movement itself. This is not to say that the correct representation of object properties must not be reactivated by visual input, prior to, or during the preshape. It has been shown that prehension movements directed at objects presented within the peripheral visual field are not only slower and less accurate; the grip formation is incomplete, the fingers do not shape properly [41]. Similarly, grasping directed at memorized objects involves larger grip apertures than grasping directed at visible objects [29].

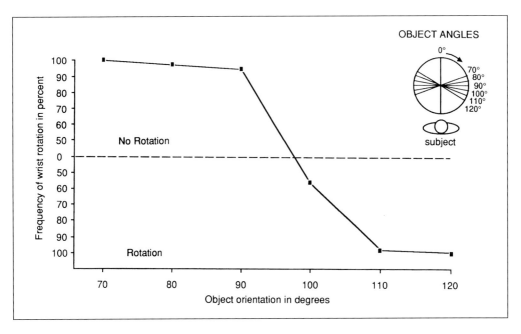

Fig. 4. Grasp preferences in normal subjects during presentation of an elongated object presented at different orientations (object orientation, in degrees of arc). The frequency (in percent of trials) of wrist rotation (pronation) was plotted for each orientation of the object. Refer to figure 5 for object shape and type of grip. From Stelmach et al. [38].

Nonvisual Aspects of Grasping

Another aspect of grip accuracy is specification of grip force. This parameter also has to be, at least partly, specified in advance, during the preshaping phase, in order for the adequate forces to be applied on the object at the onset of the grasp. Lifting an object implies a sequence of coordinated events where the grip force (to grasp the object) and the load force (to lift the object) vary in parallel. The grip force/load force ratio must exceed the slip ratio, itself determined by the coefficient of friction between the skin and the object surface. Changing the coefficient of friction (by using an object coated with sandpaper, suede or silk, for instance) changes the grip force, so that the load force remains invariant and the grip force/load force ratio increases when frictional forces decrease. By contrast, increasing the weight of the object results in an increase of both grip force and load force and in an invariant grip force/load force ratio [42].

The respective contributions of anticipatory mechanisms and of reflex adjustments to the accuracy of grip force have been extensively studied. It appears that the adaptive changes in grip force are strongly dependent on tactile afferent signals. A demonstration of this point is that adaptation of the grip force to friction disappears if the fingertips are anesthetized. The duration of the initial, isometric, phase of lifting movements (the preload phase, ca. 100 ms) is sufficient for tactile afferents from the fast adapting receptors to come into play, the latency between the onset of the slip and the change in the force ratio being in the range of 75 ms. In addition, these fast adapting receptors are very sensitive to slip signals [42, 43]. These signals may be used for updating the initial forces based on internal representation of object properties, and for sensorimotor learning. It is likely that visual cues related to object size will also be used for building this representation [see 44]. Several experiments have shown that available information about object weight, compliance, texture (e.g., based on visual size cues) can accurately determine grip and load forces in advance with respect to the grasp itself [45].

These data are critical for assessing the content of the representation that the subject has formed about the object, which expressed itself during the initial stage of the grasp (the preshape that occurs during the reach). Fingers shape in anticipation to object size and shape, the wrist rotates in anticipation to object orientation to give the optimal stability to the grasp, forces are generated which will be applied immediately at the time of contact, in order to grasp and lift the object.

Reaching and Grasping: A Goal-Dependent Coordination

Although reach and grasp can be described as separate subsystems, studies of reaching in isolation from grasping ignore many of the key aspects of its control. Similarly, studies of grasping which do not take into account the reaching component may give an incomplete picture. This is because the kinematic redundancy of the whole limb, and not only its distal segments, is exploited in building the appropriate opposition space.

The current model for explaining the coordination of actions involving simultaneously several motor components, like prehension, is that of parallel functional ensembles, characterized by specific input-output relationships, and specialized for generating each component of the action [see 22, 26, 46]. During prehension, the reaching arm movement carrying the hand to the location of the target-object is executed in parallel with finger movements which shape the hand in anticipation of the grasp. Thus, the input of the visuomotor channel specialized for grasping, for example, is tuned to visual object size, and its output is connected to distal muscles for generating a precision grip. The other channel specialized for the proximal aspect of the movement obviously must have a different structure and mode of activation. The experimental arguments suggesting that, in primates, the respective motor systems involved in reaching and in grasping movements can be considered as separate modules have been reviewed in several papers [see 47].

Time-Based Coordination

Theories involving parallel activation, however, are faced with the problem of how the different systems that are separately, and simultaneously, activated can be coordinated with each other in order to achieve the desired action. The notion that the two components of prehension might be separate movements with different modes of organization, and belonging to different levels of visual processing, should imply different timing. Yet, they must be bound to each other, so that transport of the hand and shaping of the fingers coincide in time and the reach terminates exactly at the time where the fingers come in contact with the object. Such a coordination mechanism cannot be regulated by tactile input. Activation of cutaneous afferents at the time of contact of fingers with the object would not be sufficient, in spite of the rapidity of tactile-motor loops, to account for a proper timing of prehension. By extrapolating from the Johansson and Westling data (see above), the delay of 75 ms needed for tactile signals to influence an ongoing movement means that, if the hand is still travelling at 1 m/s at the time of contact, it will pass the object location by more than 7 cm before full stop. This would not be compatible with either the degree of accuracy required for grasping, or with the observed spatiotemporal organization of the grasp.

An alternative hypothesis is that coordination between the two components pertains to a preorganized functional temporal structure. One way to assess this modality of coordination is to look for possible invariant kinematic relationships between the respective trajectories of the involved limb segments, during natural movements. It was shown by Jeannerod [27] that the time to maximum grip aperture occurred at a fixed ratio of total movement time (75–80% of movement time in most subjects). Very similar values (72–82%) were found in a sample of adult subjects studied by Von Hofsten and Rönnqvist [48]. This result was further replicated and expanded by Wallace and Weeks [28] and Wallace et al. [49], who showed that the ratio of time to maximum grip to movement time was remarkably stable in spite of large variations in movement time and speed and in spite of different initial postures of the fingers.

This temporal invariance is also preserved in situations where the 'difficulty' of the task is manipulated. Marteniuk et al [32] found prehension movements to last longer when the size of the object was smaller, that is, when the surface available for contact with the fingers was reduced. Movement time increased because the deceleration phase of reaching was longer, as it is frequently observed when total movement time changes as a function of task constraints [e.g., 50]. This finding is consistent with the fact that movement time is generally a function of task difficulty, as predicted by the Fitts' law [51]. In confirmation of this explanation, Zaal and Bootsma [52] and Bootsma et al. [53] compared movements directed at large (cylindrical) and small (oblate) objects having the same surface for positioning the fingers. As the difficulty of the task remained the same, no effect was observed on the transport component of the movements [see also 54].

The important point is that, in addition to affecting movement time, object size (or surface of contact) also affects the timing of the grip. Marteniuk et al. [32] showed that the time to maximum grip aperture was a function of task difficulty, such that maximum grip size occurred earlier for more difficult targets. Similar data were reported by Gentilucci et al. [30] and Jakobson and Goodale [55]. These results thus clearly indicate that the two components remain time-locked, and the temporal invariance of the action of grasping is preserved. Hoff and Arbib [56] have proposed a model for such time-based coordinations. This model can predict kinematic changes in either component when the other one varies. An example of such changes is provided by experiments where one of the components is 'perturbed' by suddenly changing either the position of the target object, or its apparent size after the onset of the movement [57,58].

Whole Limb Coordination during Grasping

The problem for the motor system of the hand during grasping is to build an 'opposition space' which would take into account both the shape of the object and the biomechanics of the hand. Observations like those of Stelmach et al. [38] showing that different orientations of the same object in the workspace may yield different types of grips suggest the existence of a higher order coordination mechanism which couples the different components of prehension (fig. 5). The task of the visuomotor transformation would be, first, to determine the opposition space embedded in the object to be grasped and the direction of the approach vector; and, second, to use all the available degrees of freedom of the upper limb to achieve the correct finger posture. The formation of the grasping configuration of the hand prior to contact with the object would thus be the critical factor that governs the movements of the other segments of the upper limb during the reach. Recent experiments by Desmurget et al [59] showed that the final posture of the upper limb in a prehension

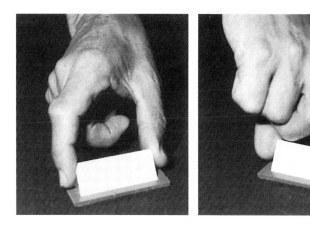

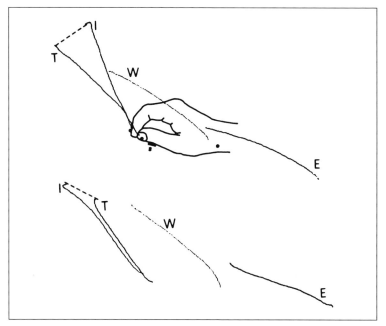

Fig. 5. Changes in whole limb configuration as a function of object orientation. An elongated object was presented at different orientations yielding different types of grip (upper photographs). On the photograph on the left, the grip involved placing the index on the left extremity of the object. Changing the orientation resulted in a grip with the index on the right extremity (photograph on the right). The lower part of the figure represents the trajectory of markers placed on the elbow (E) and wrist (W) joints and on the index (I) and thumb (T) fingertips during the first (upper row) and the second (lower row) type of movements. Dotted line represents orientation of the object. Note different trajectories of the fingers, due to the fact that the second type of movement involved wrist pronation, absent from the first type. Also note different trajectories of the elbow, due to different degrees of rotation at the glenohumeral joint. Records were made using a Selspot system, with sampling frequency at 250 Hz. From Stelmach et al. [38].

task resulted from a fixed synergy of joint positions. This result is compatible with the idea that prehension movements are programmed in joint space as a postural transition between an initial and a final limb posture. The boundaries of task variables (e.g., object orientation) within which the same final posture can be maintained still remain to be determined.

The question is therefore to know to what extent the notion of opposition space as a top-down coordination factor can be incorporated into the hypothesis of separate visuomotor channels. It is a fact that different orientations of the same object induce not only different degrees of forearm rotation, but also different degrees of rotation of the glenohumeral joint: realignment of the finger opposition space therefore activates muscles which are also used for transport. It is also true that most of the muscles involved in prehension are multifunctional: wrist pronators are also elbow flexors; muscles involved in grip formation are also involved in wrist flexion-extension, etc. (Intrinsic hand muscles may represent an exception to this rule.) The consequence is that, during prehension, the same torque may be applied at the same time at different joints by contraction of the same muscle. Because the moment of inertia of components is different (it is smaller for the more distal ones) the same torque will produce different acceleration profiles at each joint. The timing of the overall movement will therefore be imposed by that of the transport component which has the greater inertia. Variations in amplitude of the other components, which require less time, will be possible within this temporal frame. Lacquaniti and Soechting [60] have used this reasoning to explain the apparent lack of forearm rotation coupling with shoulder and elbow flexion-extension. This might explain why, in the observations of Stelmach et al., [38] grasping movements with or without rotation of the wrist had the same duration. Movement duration would represent a time frame within which each given component can vary without affecting the others. If temporal constraints are imposed on the task, as in making rapid movement or in making corrections, the duration of the movement (and, more specifically, of its deceleration phase) will have to increase for preserving the temporal scaling between components.

References

1   Bell C: The Hand: Its Mechanism and Vital Endowments as Evincing Design. Bridgewater Treatise, IV. London, Pickering, 1833.
2   Berkeley G: A New Theory of Vision. London, Dent, 1734; new ed 1972.
3   Napier JR: The prehensile movements of the human hand. J Bone Joint Surg [B] 1956;38:902–913.
4   Elliott JM, Connolly KJ: A classification of manipulative hand movements. Dev Med Child Neurol 1984;26: 283–296.
5   Heffner R, Masterton B: Variation in form of the pyramidal tract and its relationship to digital dexterity. Brain Behav Evol 1975;12:161–200.
6   Napier JR: Prehensility and opposability in the hands of primates. Symp Zool Soc (Lond) 1961;5:115–132.
7   Susman RL: Hand of *Paranthropus robustus* from member 1, Swartkrans. Science 1988;240:781–784.
8   Napier JR: Studies of the hands of living primates. Proc Zool Soc (Lond) 1960;134:647–657.
9   Grew WC: Why is ape tool-use so confusing? In Standen V, Foley RA (eds): The Behavioural Ecology of Humans and Other Mammals. Oxford, Blackwell, 1989.
10   Christel M: Grasping techniques and hand preferences in *Hominoidea*; in Preuschoft H, Chivers DJ (eds): Hands of Primates. New York, Springer, 1993, pp 91–108.
11   Christel M: Greiftechniken und Handpräferenzen verschiedener catarrhiner Primaten beim Aufnehmen kleiner Objekte; Inaug Diss, Freie Universität Berlin, 1993.
12   Jouffroy FK: Primate hands and the human hand. The tool of tools; in Berthelet A, Chavaillon J (eds): The Use of Tools by Human and Non-Human Primates. Oxford, Oxford University Press, 1993, pp 6–33.
13   Fragaszy DM: Preliminary quantitative studies of prehension in squirrel monkeys (*Saimiri sciureus*). Brain Behav Evol 1983;23:81–92.
14   Tower SS: Pyramidal lesion in the monkey. Brain 1940;63:36–90.

15 Passingham RE, Perry H, Wilkinson F: Failure to develop a precision grip in monkeys with unilateral neocortical lesions made in infancy. Brain Res 1978;145:410–414.

16 Chapman E, Wiesendanger M: Recovery of function following unilateral lesions of the bulbar pyramid in the monkey. Electroencephalogr Clin Neurophysiol 1982;53:374–38.

17 Bortoff GA, Strick PL: Corticospinal terminations in two new-world primates. Further evidence that corticomo-toneuronal connections provide part of the manual substrate for manual dexterity. J Neurosci 1993;13:5105–5118.

18 Phillips CG: Movements of the Hand. Liverpool, Liverpool University Press, 1985.

19 Jeannerod M: The representing brain. Neural correlates of motor intention and imagery. Behav Brain Sci 1994; 17:187–245.

20 Sakata H, Shibutani H, Kawano K, Harrington TL: Neural mechanisms of space vision in the parietal association cortex of the monkey. Vision Res 1985;25:453–463.

21 Taira M, Mine S, Georgopoulos AP, Murata A, Sakata H: Parietal cortex neurons of the monkey related to the visual guidance of hand movements. Exp Brain Res 1990;83:29–36.

22 Arbib MA: Perceptual structures and distributed motor control; in Brooks VB (ed): Handbook of Physiology, Section I: The Nervous System, vol 2: Motor Control. Baltimore, Williams & Wilkins, 1981, pp 1449–1480.

23 Arbib MA: Schemas for the temporal organization of behavior. Hum Neurobiol 1985;4:63–72.

24 Iberall T, Arbib MA: Schemas for the control of hand movements: An essay on cortical localization; in Goodale MA (ed): Vision and Action: The Control of Grasping, Norwood, Ablex, 1990, pp 204–242.

25 Iberall T, Bingham G, Arbib MA: Opposition space as a structuring concept for the analysis of skilled hand movements. Exp Brain Res 1986(suppl 15):158–173.

26 Jeannerod M: Intersegmental coordination during reaching at natural visual objects; in Long J, Baddeley A (eds): Attention and Performance. IX. Hillsdale, Erlbaum, 1981, pp 153–168.

27 Jeannerod M: The timing of natural prehension movements. J Mot Behav 1984;16:235–254.

28 Wallace SA, Weeks DL: Temporal constraints in the control of prehensive movements. J Mot Behav 1988;20: 81–105.

29 Wing AM, Turton A, Fraser C: Grasp size and accuracy of approach in reaching. J Mot Behav 1986;18: 245–260.

30 Gentilucci M, Castiello U, Corradini ML, Scarpa M, Umiltà C, Rizzolatti G: Influence of different types of grasping on the transport component of prehension movements. Neuropsychologia 1991;29:361–378.

31 Wing AM, Fraser C: The contribution of the thumb to reaching movements. Q J Exp Psychol 1983;35A: 297–309.

32 Marteniuk RG, Leavitt JL, MacKenzie CL, Athenes S: Functional relationships between grasp and transport components in a prehension task. Hum Mov Sci 1990;9:149–176.

33 Jeannerod M, Decety J, Michel F: Impairment of grasping movements following a bilateral posterior parietal lesion. Neuropsychologia 1994;32:369–380.

34 Jeannerod M, Decety J: The accuracy of visuomotor transformation. An investigation into the mechanisms of visual recognition of objects; in Goodale M (ed): Vision and Action. The Control of Grasping. Norwood, Ablex, 1990, pp 33–48.

35 Ekman G, Junge K: Psychophysical relations in visual perception of length, area and volume. Scand J Psychol 1961;2:1–10.

36 Stevens SS, Guirao M: Subjective scaling of length and area and matching of length to loudness and brightness. J Exp Psychol 1963;66:177–186.

37 Teghtsoonian M: The judgement of size. Am J Psychol 1965;76:392–402.

38 Stelmach GE, Castiello U, Jeannerod M: Orienting the finger opposition space during prehension movements. J Mot Behav 1994;26:178–186.

39 Rosenbaum DA, Marchak F, Barnes HJ, Vaughan J, Slotta JD, Jorgensen MJ: Constraints for action selection. Overhand versus underhand grips; in Jeannerod M (ed): Motor Representation and Control, Attention and Performance. XIII. Hillsdale Erlbaum, 1990, pp 321–342.

40 Rosenbaum DA, Jorgensen MJ: Planning macroscopic aspects of manual control. Hum Mov Sci 1992;11:61–69.

41 Sivak B, MacKenzie CL: The contribution of peripheral vision and central vision to prehension; in Proteau L, Elliott D (eds): Vision and Motor Control. Amsterdam, Elsevier, 1992.

42 Johansson RS, Westling G: Signals in tactile afferents from the fingers eliciting adaptive motor responses during precision grip. Exp Brain Res 1987;66:141–154.

43 Westling G, Johansson RS: Factors influencing the force control during precision grip. Exp Brain Res 1984; 53:277–284.

44 Johansson RS, Westling G: Coordinated isometric muscles commands adequately and erroneously programmed for the weight during lifting task with precision grip. Exp Brain Res 1988;71:59–71.

45 Gordon AM, Forssberg H, Johansson RS, Westling G: Visual size cues in the programming of manipulative forces during precision grip. Exp Brain Res 1991;83:477–482.

46 Jeannerod M, Biguer B: Visuomotor mechanisms in reaching within extrapersonal space; in Ingle D, Goodale MA, Mansfield R (eds): Advances in the Analysis of Visual Behavior. Boston, MIT Press, 1982, pp 387–409.

47 Jeannerod M, Arbib MA, Rizzolatti G, Sakata H: Grasping objects. The cortical mechanisms of visuomotor transformation. Trends Neurosci 1995;18:214–320.

48 Von Hofsten C, Rönnqvist L: Preparation for grasping an object: A developmental study. J Exp Psychol 1988; 14:610–621.

49   Wallace SA, Weeks DL, Kelso JAS: Temporal constraints in reaching and grasping behavior. Hum Mov Sci 1990;9:69–93.
50   Marteniuk RG, MacKenzie CL, Jeannerod M, Athenes S, Dugas C: Constraints on human arm movement trajectories. Can J Psychol 1987;41:365–378.
51   Fitts PM: The information capacity of the human motor system in controlling the amplitude of movement. J Exp Psychol 1954;47:381–39.
52   Zaal FT, Bootsma RJ: Accuracy demands in natural prehension. Hum Mov Sci 1993;12:339–345.
53   Bootsma RJ, Marteniuk RG, MacKenzie CL, Zaal FT: The speed-accuracy trade-off in manual prehension: Effect of movement amplitude, object size and object width on kinematic characteristics. Exp Brain Res 1994; 98:535–541.
54   Chieffi S, Gentilucci M: Coordination between the transport and the grasp component during prehension movements. Exp Brain Res 1993;94:471–47.
55   Jakobson LS, Goodale MA: Factors affecting higher-order movement planning: A kinematic analysis of human prehension. Exp Brain Res 1991;86:199–208.
56   Hoff B, Arbib MA: Models of trajectory formation and temporal interaction of reach and grasp. J Mot Behav 1993;25:175–192.
57   Paulignan Y, MacKenzie CL, Marteniuk RG, Jeannerod M: Selective perturbation of visual input during prehension movements. 1. The effects of changing object position. Exp Brain Res 1991;83:502–512.
58   Paulignan Y, Jeannerod M, MacKenzie CL, Marteniuk RG: Selective perturbation of visual input during prehension movements. 2. Effects of changing object size. Exp Brain Res 1991;87:407–420.
59   Desmurget M, Prablanc C, Rossetti Y, Arzi M, Paulignan Y, Urquizar C, Mignot JC: Postural and synergic control for three-dimensional movements of reaching and grasping. J Neurophysiol 1995;74:905–910.
60   Lacquaniti F, Soechting J: Coordination of arm and wrist motion during a reaching task. J Neurosci 1982;2: 399–408.

Dr. Marc Jeannerod, Vision et Motricité, INSERM U94,
16 avenue du Doyen Lépine, F–69500 Bron (France)

Hepp-Reymond M-C, Marini G (eds): Perspectives of Motor Behavior and Its Neural Basis.
Basel, Karger, 1997, pp 33–43

....

Effect of Inactivation of the Hand Representation of the Primary and Supplementary Motor Cortical Areas on Precision Grip Performance in Monkeys

Eric M. Rouiller, Xiao-Hong Yu, Aldo Tempini

Institute of Physiology, University of Fribourg, Switzerland

In primates, four principal zones of the frontal cortex are commonly recognized as contributing directly to the control of hand movements: the primary motor cortex (M1 or area 4), the supplementary motor area (SMA or mesial part of area 6), the premotor cortex (lateral part of area 6) and the cingulate motor area (areas 23 and 24). A large zone of M1 is involved in the selection of distal muscles of the contralateral forelimb, as shown by intracortical microstimulation (ICMS) eliciting wrist and/or finger movements [e.g., 1–7]. A rostral (pre-SMA or area F6) and a caudal (SMA-proper or area F3) subdivisions have been distinguished in SMA [8, 9]. A distal hand representation has been found in SMA-proper, but whether a second hand representation is present in pre-SMA remains unclear [9–11]. M1 is the origin of corticospinal axons, which make in primates direct contacts with cervical motoneurons [12]. This corticomotoneuronal system is believed to subserve the ability to perform independent, finely controlled, movements of the fingers [13], such as the precision grip used to pick an object between the thumb and the index finger [see Jeannerod, chap. 2]. Surgical lesion of the M1 hand representation in monkeys dramatically affects precision grip ability [14]. A contingent of corticospinal neurons also has its origin in SMA [15, 16], and there is some preliminary evidence that the axons of some of them may also contact the motoneurons [17, 18]. The question thus arises whether SMA, in cooperation with M1, is contributing to the control of the precision grip.

Following unilateral surgical lesion of SMA, a clear deficit in precision grip was observed up to 7 days postoperation [19]. However, the interpretation of lesion data has a number of limitations, in particular the presence of long-term plastic changes and development of compensatory strategies. Regional reversible inactivations by pharmacological or cooling methods have been introduced to minimize these difficulties. The aim of the present study was first to quantify in monkeys the precision grip deficit associated to inactivation of the hand representation of M1 and, second, by comparison to investigate the effect of SMA inactivation. Previous transient inactivation of SMA by cooling showed that single joint wrist movements or key press movements were not impaired [11, 20]. It is however not certain whether this would be true for the multijoint precision grip, which

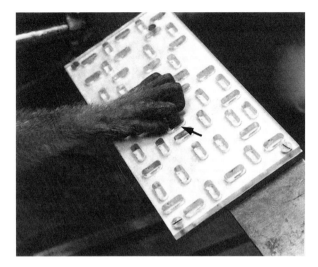

Fig. 1. Behavioral set-up and illustration of picking up the food morsel between the tips of index finger and the thumb from a vertical slot (arrow).

cannot be considered as a simple movement. Precision grip requires the coordination of a large number of muscles [21, 22], as well as effective inhibitory processes to move one or two single digits without moving the other fingers [11].

Methods

Two monkeys (*Macaca fascicularis*) were trained to perform daily a precision grip task (fig. 1) in a modified version of a standard test [23], using a plastic board ($20 \cdot 10$ cm) containing 50 rectangular slots (15 mm long, 6 mm wide and 6 mm deep), 25 oriented vertically and 25 horizontally. The monkeys were trained during 5–15 days to pick up with dexterity a piece of food (cookie) in each slot with the left or the right hand. After training, the behavioral performance was assessed during 30 daily sessions, by counting the number of food morsels successfully retrieved with the left hand during 60 s. When the food morsel was dropped during transport to the mouth, the trial was not considered as successful, because it also reflects a deficit in the precision grip. The present report is restricted to the performance of the left hand, because the 2 monkeys were subjected to a neonatal lesion of the hand representation in the left M1, while the right M1 was intact. To verify that the lesion in the left M1 did not affect the performance of the left hand, a third intact monkey was tested in the same task and exhibited a comparable score for the two hands (Mann-Whitney test, NS). More important, the scores obtained in the two neonatally lesioned monkeys with their left hand were similar to the scores of the control monkey (Mann-Whitney test, NS).

Typically (fig. 1), the monkey first inserted the index finger in the slot and then brought the thumb into opposition, to pick up the food morsel out of the slot, as previously described in detail [19]. The task was more difficult for the horizontal than the vertical slots, because the monkey had to rotate the arm to access the horizontal slots. At the end of the behavioral evaluation (scores of the left hand established in 30 daily sessions), the monkey was anesthetized (pentobarbital, 30 mg/kg) and a chronic metallic chamber was implanted, allowing access to M1 and SMA on both sides and fixation of the head. The somatotopy of M1 was established by ICMS (fig. 2), as previously reported [2, 16, 24]. The ICMS parameters were the following: 36 ms duration trains of 12 electric pulses (0.2 ms) at 330 Hz, presented once every 2 s. ICMS was performed in daily sessions lasting 1 h, during which

Table 1. Summary of the characteristics of the inactivation sessions performed on monkeys 1 and 2

Session	Monkey	Cortical area inactivated	Total volume of lidocaine infused, µl	Number of sites of infusion
1	1	M1-R	10	6
2	2	M1-R	18	9
3	2	M1-R	8	6
4	1	SMA-R[1]	6	4
5	1	SMA-L[1]	6	4
6	2	SMA + pre-SMA bilaterally	14	14
7	2	SMA + pre-SMA bilaterally	14	14
8	2	SMA-R + pre-SMA-R	7	7

Session 7 was a repetition of session 6, 1 week later. The results were the same (see text).

[1] Infusion of lidocaine restricted to the caudal part of SMA, corresponding to SMA-proper.

4–10 vertical electrode penetrations were made. From the pial surface, on a distance of 8–10 mm along each penetration, the ICMS effect and threshold were assessed every 500 µm. Two to 3 months later, a second training period of 10 (monkey 1) and 27 (monkey 2) days was necessary to habituate the animal to perform the food morsel retrieval task with the head fixed. The animals were not food deprived, but the behavioral testing represented their first daily meal followed by additional food as reinforcement.

The behavioral tests were pursued on a daily basis for several weeks. During this period, for each monkey, an inactivation session took place once a week. On that day, the animal first performed the behavioral task (control scores), and then a given cortical region was reversibly inactivated by infusing the local anesthetic lidocaine (4% solution in saline), as previously described [e.g. 25–27]. Lidocaine was injected by pressure using a 10-µl Hamilton microsyringe. Five to 10 min after injection, the task was repeated to assess the effect of the inactivation. Thirty to 60 min later, when the action of lidocaine faded out, the motor task was repeated a third time to check that the animal recovered from the transient inactivation. In a given inactivation session, lidocaine was injected either in the hand area of M1 on the right side (M1-R), or in SMA on the right side (SMA-R), or in SMA on the left side (SMA-L). In two particular sessions on monkey 2, to test the effect of the simultaneous inactivation of both SMAs, SMA-R was inactivated first, followed immediately by inactivation of SMA-L (table 1).

In session 1 (table 1), M1-R was inactivated in monkey 1: a volume of 1.5–2.0 µl of lidocaine was injected in each of 6 sites, where ICMS elicited movements of fingers or wrist at low threshold (fig. 2). In two other experiments in monkey 2 (table 1: inactivation sessions 2 and 3), lidocaine (1–2 µl) was injected at each of 6 or 9 sites in M1-R (in the fingers and wrist representations as determined by ICMS). To inject lidocaine, the Hamilton microsyringe was oriented vertically (as the electrode tracks for ICMS) and placed on the pial surface exactly at the same coordinates as the corresponding electrode penetration along which ICMS elicited distal movements (thumb, fingers or wrist). As opposed to electrode penetrations perpendicular to the pial surface, different movements may be elicited by ICMS at different depths along vertical penetrations (for instance elbow, wrist, fingers). To avoid infusion of lidocaine in cortical representations more proximal than the wrist (e.g. elbow, shoulder), the depth of the microsyringe with respect to the pial surface was also matched to the depth of the

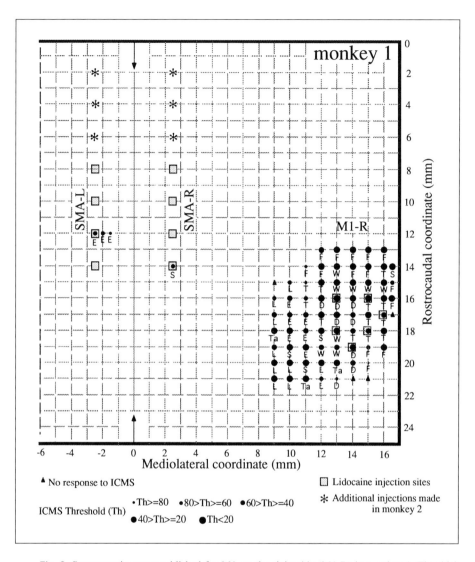

Fig. 2. Somatotopic map established for M1 on the right side (M1-R) in monkey 1. The thick line represents the right half of the chronically implanted metallic chamber. The filled symbols represent the location on the brain surface of electrode penetrations for ICMS. The body territories activated are indicated as follows: D = digits (fingers 2–5); E = elbow; F = face; L = leg; S = shoulder; T = thumb; Ta = tail; W = wrist. The threshold (Th) to obtain the ICMS effects is indicated by the size of the symbols (see below graph). ICMS points where lidocaine has been injected are indicated by shaded rectangles. In SMA, the same rectangles indicate the location of lidocaine injections. The two vertical arrows (at mediolateral coordinate zero) represent the midline, in between the two hemispheres.

sites at which distal (fingers, wrist) ICMS effects were obtained at low currents (generally < 10 μA). The precise matching of the ICMS electrode and microsyringe penetrations provided then confidence that lidocaine was infused at a site that belongs to the hand representation. Hand representations mixed with or nearby to more proximal territories (e.g. elbow) were not selected as targets for lidocaine infusion.

Table 2. Behavioral scores of the left hand in the food morsel retrieval test, measured during a series of several consecutive sessions[1], preceding inactivation experiments

	Monkey 1		Monkey 2	
	mean score	SD	mean score	SD
Vertical slots	20.3	2.7	18.6	1.8
Horizontal slots	16.2	2.7	18.6	1.8
Total	36.5	5.4	32.5	2.4

[1] The number of daily sessions was 10 for monkey 1 and 27 for monkey 2. These scores are to be compared with the scores displayed in the leftmost three bins of figures 3 and 4, and provide an estimate of the variability across sessions (SDs).

In SMA, the location of the arm representation was roughly established bilaterally based on elbow or shoulder movements elicited by ICMS (fig. 2), to determine the appropriate mediolateral coordinate. Two distinct inactivation sessions were performed on monkey 1 to inactivate SMA unilaterally: in the first one (session 4), lidocaine (1.5 μl) was injected in SMA-R 4 mm below pial surface in each of four penetrations along the rostrocaudal axis, covering SMA-proper (fig. 2); in the other SMA experiment (inactivation session 5), lidocaine (same volume) was infused in corresponding points in SMA-L (four penetrations along the rostrocaudal axis, see fig. 2). Two lidocaine microinjections were positioned rostrally with respect to the sites where ICMS elicited movements of the elbow or shoulder (fig. 2); therefore, the inactivated regions included also the hand representation located rostrally to the elbow and shoulder areas, according to the somatotopic map of SMA [10, 28, 29]. In monkey 2, two inactivation experiments (table1: sessions 6 and 7) were performed to inactivate SMA bilaterally. In both SMA-R and SMA-L, lidocaine was injected in four penetrations at the same locations as in monkey 1 and in three additional penetrations to include pre-SMA (see in fig. 2): in each penetration 1.0 μl was infused at each of two sites, 5 and 3 mm below the pial surface, respectively. Finally, also in monkey 2, microinjections were made in SMA and pre-SMA unilaterally, on the right side (table 1: inactivation session 8). The characteristics of the inactivation sessions (volume of lidocaine, location, number of sites of infusion) performed on monkeys 1 and 2 are summarized in table 1.

Results

Inactivation Experiments in Monkey 1

The stable level in precision grip performance was determined on the basis of measurements made several days before the inactivation experiments (table 2). The effects of inactivation of M1 or SMA-R or SMA-L on the performance of the left hand are illustrated in figure 3 for monkey 1 (data derived from inactivation sessions 1, 4 and 5; see table 1). As expected, the scores before injection were in the range of those listed in table 2. Five minutes after injection of lidocaine in M1-R, the total score of the left hand decreased by 75% (fig. 3A). The deficit was more pronounced for the horizontal slots (0% retrieved). By means of a global grip movement (flexion of all fingers at the same time), the animal could pick up the food morsel in only 8 vertical slots (fig. 3A): the digits 3–5 frequently contacted adjacent slots interfering with retrieval from the slot aimed by the monkey with

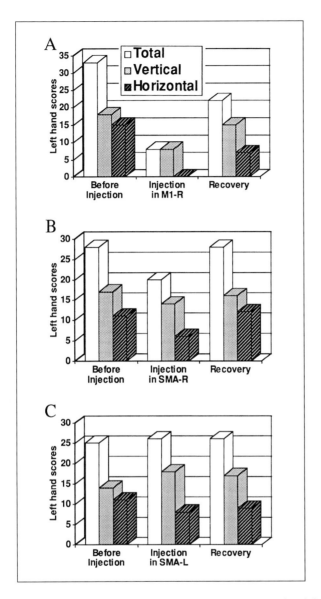

Fig. 3. Behavioral scores (number of food morsels retrieved during 60 s) with the left hand for monkey 1, before and after injection of lidocaine in M1 (**A**), in SMA-R (**B**) or in SMA-L (**C**).

the index finger. Thirty minutes after injection, a partial but significant recovery was observed (fig. 3A).

The effect of unilateral inactivation of SMA-proper was investigated in monkey 1, in two experiments in which SMA was infused with lidocaine on the right side (table 1: SMA-R, session 4) or on the left side (table 1: SMA-L, session 5). A moderate decrease of the left hand performance was noticed after inactivation of SMA-R (fig. 3B). The deficit was however qualitatively different, and involved more the proximal component of the arm

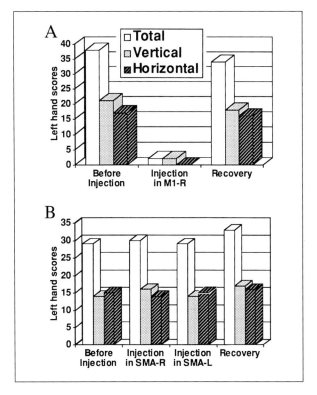

Fig. 4. Behavioral scores (number of food morsels retrieved during 60 s) with the left hand for monkey 2, before and after injection of lidocaine in M1-R (**A**) or in SMA bilaterally (**B**).

movement (reaching) than the precision grip itself. The recovery was complete (fig. 3B). The deficit related to the inactivation of SMA-R in monkey 1 (fig. 3B) can be considered as relatively minor because the difference with the scores obtained before injection or after recovery (fig. 3B) are only slightly larger than the standard deviations obtained for this animal in the preliminary tests in absence of inactivation (table 2). Inactivation of SMA-L had no effect on the performance of the left hand (fig. 3C).

Inactivation Experiments in Monkey 2

In monkey 2, inactivation of M1-R also induced a dramatic deficit of the precision grip performance (fig. 4A; see also table 1: inactivation session 2), which was even more pronounced than in monkey 1, with a decrease of 90% in the total score for the left hand. Again, no food morsel was retrieved from the horizontal slots. In a few trials, the monkey picked up the food morsel from a vertical slot using the global grip, but sometimes dropped it during the transport to the mouth (such trials were considered as unsuccessful). Thirty minutes after injection, recovery was almost complete (fig. 4A). Inactivation of M1-R was repeated in monkey 2, but the total volume of lidocaine infused and the number of sites of delivery were smaller (table 1: inactivation session 3). There was again a dramatic deficit of the left hand in the precision grip task: before inactivation, the vertical and horizontal

---

scores were 19 and 14 and, after lidocaine infusion, these scores dropped to 5 and 0, respectively.

Movement-related potentials and functional imaging data suggest that SMA on both hemispheres are often engaged simultaneously [30, 31]. The protocol was modified accordingly in monkey 2 in order to inactivate both SMAs during the same session (table 1: inactivation session 6). Furthermore, as compared to monkey 1, additional infusions of lidocaine were aimed more rostrally, in order to include pre-SMA (fig. 2). Lidocaine was first injected in SMA-R and the test performed 5 min later showed no deficit (fig. 4B). Lidocaine was then injected immediately in SMA-L, to generate a simultaneous inactivation of SMA in each hemisphere; again, no deficit was observed 5 minutes after injection in SMA-L (fig. 4B). One week later, the same protocol of lidocaine infusion in SMA-R and SMA-L (including pre-SMA on both sides) was repeated (table 1: inactivation session 7); once more, no deficit was observed in relation to inactivation of SMA-R and SMA-L simultaneously.

The comparison of the results obtained in the 2 monkeys showed a similar dramatic deficit after inactivation of M1: the behavioral score reflecting precision grip ability dropped by 75–90%. In contrast, slightly different results were obtained in the two monkeys after inactivation of SMA-R (figs. 3B, 4B). For that reason, inactivation of SMA-R was repeated in monkey 2 (table 1: inactivation session 8), confirming the absence of deficit shown in figure 4B. The effect observed in monkey 1 for SMA-R inactivation is close to the inter-session variability (see SDs in table 2). In addition, the deficits concerned essentially the wrist and more proximal muscles. Therefore, it seems reasonable to conclude that inactivation of SMA-R and/or SMA-L did not affect significantly the precision grip ability of the left hand, in contrast to M1-R, as judged by the precision grip performance. However, one cannot rule out that SMA may play a role in the control of subtle parameters of the precision grip, such as precise trajectory, force, velocity, etc., which were not measured in the present experiment.

Discussion

The present study confirms the established notion that the hand representation of M1 plays a major role in the control of fine movements performed independently with the fingers [14], such as the precision grip. Although there are preliminary indications that SMA may also have a direct access to the cervical motoneurons [17, 18], it does not seem to be a substitute for M1 when this cortical region is made dysfunctional by a pharmacological agent. However, this does not imply that SMA cannot substitute M1 if the M1 dysfunction were prolonged or permanent. One possibility is that corticomotoneuronal connections originating from SMA might be present [17, 18], but may be functional only after a period of adaptation following a lesion of M1. This idea is consistent with the occurrence of single neuron activities in SMA associated to a well-practiced movement, following surgical lesion of M1 [32]. In the present experimental paradigm, the inactivation of M1 is probably too short lasting to induce such changes.

In contrast, inactivation of SMA either unilaterally or bilaterally did not affect precision grip performance significantly (fig. 3B,C, 4B). This means that SMA (in fact SMA-proper as well as pre-SMA) contributes little, if at all, to the control of the precision grip as judged by the behavioral performance. This result contrasts with the observation of a significant deficit in precision grip performance 7 days after surgical lesion of SMA [19]. Most likely the surgical lesion involved a larger cortical territory, possibly encroaching on cingulate motor areas and the corpus callosum, as compared to the limited territories inactivated by application of lidocaine [25]. Moreover, the inactivation lasted only a few minutes in the present case (lidocaine) while the surgical lesions of Brinkman were permanent. Another reason for the differences with the study of Brinkman [19] is that a surgical lesion does not exclusively affect the area removed, but more generally induces dramatic changes in the connectivity among the various motor cortical areas and with subcortical centers. As a consequence, the observed deficit may not be related exclusively to the area that was removed but also to other areas which became disconnected and in which anterograde and retrograde degenerations took place. Thus, because of the strong interconnections between M1 and SMA [e.g. 10, 33, 34], one might expect that the surgical lesion of the SMA performed by Brinkman [19] indirectly also affected M1. Another difference between pharmacological transient inactivation and surgical permanent lesions, in the view of the multiple motor cortical areas working in a collaborative manner (via their multiple interconnections), is that a surgical lesion will first disrupt that circuit and later lead to a reorganization of the network. In contrast, a short lasting pharmacological inactivation transiently interrupts the connectivity between the multiple motor cortical areas but a rearrangement of the circuit is not likely to occur during such a short time.

In the same line, the present results based on transient inactivation of the SMA apparently differ from previous observations derived from ablation of the SMA [35]. These authors reported the appearance after unilateral SMA ablation of a contralateral 'forced grasping'. This is a pathological prehension presenting the two following characteristics: grasping can easily be elicited by cutaneous stimulation of the hand, and once grasping has occurred the animal is unable to release the object [35]. In the present experiments of reversible inactivation of the SMA, tactile stimulation of the hand was not tested and the animal did not exhibit any inability to release the food morsel from the grasp when bringing it to the mouth. However, forced grasping does not systematically appear following a lesion restricted to the SMA: there is evidence that forced grasping is more prominent when the lesion included not only the SMA, but also more lateral regions of area 6 [35]. In the study of Smith et al. [35], the ablation was clearly not restricted to the SMA, encroaching more lateral territories. In contrast, the lidocaine injections performed here most likely should not include territories more lateral than the SMA, if one considers the estimations of the extent of the reversible inactivation of the cerebral cortex, made by Martin [25] after comparable microinjections of lidocaine in the rat. Finally, although the study of Smith et al. [35] and the present one both investigated the precision grip, the movements tested were not the same: the food morsel retrieval task tested here is clearly different from compressing a force transducer between thumb and index fingers [35]. This may also explain in part the different results obtained in the two studies, although the differences between surgical lesion and reversible pharmacological inactivation are likely to play a more prominent role.

Although precision grip is not a simple movement [11, 21, 22], the present study shows that it was not affected by inactivation of SMA, a result reminiscent of the absence of effect of SMA cooling on single joint movements [11, 20]. Possibly more relevant than the degree of complexity of a movement is the fact that the precision grip belongs to the primate natural repertoire (e.g. grooming). In addition, because of the daily repetition of the tests, the precision grip became for our monkeys extremely well practiced, if not overtrained. The absence of effect of SMA inactivation on the relatively automatic precision grip appears consistent with the idea that SMA is more involved in the preparatory phase and the initiation of more complex (multijoint, sequential) movements rather than in the movement execution [36, 37]. This is consistent with reports of single neuron activities in SMA which were associated to a motor task, but progressively disappeared when the task became overtrained [32]. Inactivation of SMA might then have been more effective on precision grip during the training period. However, PET data in humans suggest that SMA is more active during performance of a prelearned task than during new learning [38]. A recent study showed that the activity of SMA neurons was exclusively related to a specific movement within a sequence, but only when it was performed in a particular order, in contrast to M1 neurons [39]. Transient inactivation of SMA may thus affect more the organization of a sequence of movements than the natural precision grip.

Conclusion

In conclusion, the present work demonstrates that unilateral transient inactivation of M1 severely affected the precision grip performance of the contralateral hand in monkeys, confirming previous lesion data [14]. In sharp contrast, reversible inactivation of SMA (unilateral or bilateral) did not significantly impair this performance, in disagreement with the deficit previously reported after a surgical SMA lesion [19]. The present data are consistent with the idea that SMA does not play a major role in the control of such overtrained movements or of movements belonging to the primate natural repertoire and might contribute more to the learning and/or execution of more complex movements, in particular sequences of movements.

Acknowledgements

The present work was supported by the Swiss National Science Foundation (grants 3130-025138, 31-28572.90, 31-43422.95). The authors thank V. Moret for technical assistance, J. Corpataux and B. Morandi for taking care of the monkeys in the animal room.

References

1   Asanuma H, Rosén I: Topographical organization of cortical efferent zones projecting to distal forelimb muscles in the monkey. Exp Brain Res 1972;14:243–256.
2   Sessle BJ, Wiesendanger M: Structural and functional definition of the motor cortex in the monkey (*Macaca fascicularis*). J Physiol (Lond) 1982;323:245–265.
3   Lemon R: The output map of the primate motor cortex. Trends Neurosci 1988;11:501–506.
4   Schieber MH: How might the motor cortex individuate movements? Trends Neurosci 1990;13:440–445.
5   Schmidt EM, McIntosh JS: Microstimulation mapping of precentral cortex during trained movements. J Neurophysiol 1990;64:1668–1682.
6   Huntley GW, Jones EG: Relationship of intrinsic connections to forelimb movement representations in monkey motor cortex: A correlative anatomic and physiological study. J Neurophysiol 1991;66:390–413.
7   Donoghue JP, Leibovic S, Sanes JN: Organization of the forelimb area in squirrel monkey motor cortex: Representation of digit, wrist, and elbow muscles. Exp Brain Res 1992;89:1–19.
8   Luppino G, Matelli M, Camarda RM, Gallese V, Rizzolatti G: Multiple representations of body movements in mesial area 6 and the adjacent cingulate cortex: An intracortical microstimulation study in the macaque monkey. J Comp Neurol 1991;311:463–482.
9   Matsuzaka Y, Aizawa H, Tanji J: A motor area rostral to the supplementary motor area (presupplementary motor area) in the monkey: Neuronal activity during a learned motor task. J Neurophysiol 1992;68:653–662.
10   Wiesendanger M: Recent developments in studies of the supplementary motor area of primates. Rev Physiol Biochem Pharmacol 1986;103:1–59.

11 Tanji J: The supplementary motor area in the cerebral cortex. Neurosci Res 1994;19:251–268.

12 Lawrence DG, Porter R, Redman SJ: Corticomotoneuronal synapses in the monkey: Light microscopic localization upon motoneurons of intrinsic muscles of the hand. J Comp Neurol 1985;232:499–510.

13 Lemon RN: Cortical control of the primate hand. Exp Physiol 1993;78: 263–301.

14 Passingham RE, Perry VH, Wilkinson F: The long-term effects of removal of sensorimotor cortex in infant and adult rhesus monkeys. Brain 1983;106:675–705.

15 Dum RP, Strick PL: The origin of corticospinal projections from the premotor areas in the frontal lobe. J Neurosci 1991;11:667–689.

16 Rouiller EM, Babalian A, Kazennikov O, Moret V, Yu X-H, Wiesendanger M: Transcallosal connections of the distal forelimb representations of the primary and supplementary motor cortical areas in macaque monkeys. Exp Brain Res 1994;102:227–243.

17 Rouiller EM, Moret V, Tanné J, Boussaoud D: Evidence for direct connections between the hand representation of the supplementary motor area and cervical motoneurons in the macaque monkey. Eur J Neurosci 1996;8: 1055–1059.

18 Rouiller EM: Multiple hand representations in the motor cortical areas; in Wing A, Haggard P, Flanagan R (eds): Hand and Brain: The Neurophysiology and Psychology of Hand Function. New York, Academic Press, 1996.

19 Brinkman C: Supplementary motor area of the monkey's cerebral cortex: Short- and long-term deficits after unilateral ablation and the effects of subsequent callosal section. J Neurosci 1984;4:918–929.

20 Schmidt EM, Porter R, McIntosh JS: The effects of cooling supplementary motor area and midline cerebral cortex on neuronal responses in area 4 of monkeys. Electroencephalogr Clin Neurophysiol Electromyogr Motor Control 1992;85:61–71.

21 Maier MA, Hepp-Reymond MC: EMG activation patterns during force production in precision grip. I. Contribution of 15 finger muscles to isometric force. Exp Brain Res 1995;103:108–122.

22 Maier MA, Hepp-Reymond MC: EMG activation patterns during force production in precision grip. II. Muscular synergies in the spatial and temporal domain. Exp Brain Res 1995;103:123–136.

23 Brinkman J, Kuypers HGJM: Cerebral control of contralateral and ipsilateral arm, hand and finger movements in the split-brain rhesus monkey. Brain 1973;96:653–674.

24 Rouiller EM, Liang F, Babalian A, Moret V, Wiesendanger M: Cerebellothalamocortical and pallidothalamocortical projections to the primary and supplementary motor cortical areas: A multiple tracing study in macaque monkeys. J Comp Neurol 1994;345:185–213.

25 Martin JH: Autoradiographic estimation of the extent of reversible inactivation produced by microinjection of lidocaine and muscimol in the rat. Neurosci Lett 1991;127:160–164.

26 Martin JH, Ghez C: Impairments in reaching during reversible inactivation of the distal forelimb representation of the motor cortex in the cat. Neurosci Lett 1991;133:61–64.

27 Martin JH, Cooper SE, Ghez C: Differential effects of local inactivation within motor cortex and red nucleus on performance of an elbow task in the cat. Exp Brain Res 1993;94:418–428.

28 Macpherson JM, Marangoz C, Miles TS, Wiesendanger M: Microstimulation of the supplementary motor area in the awake monkey. Exp Brain Res 1982;45:410–416.

29 Mitz AR, Wise SP: The somatotopic organization of the supplementary motor area: Intracortical microstimulation mapping. J Neurophysiol 1987;7:1010–1021.

30 Colebatch JG, Deiber MP, Passingham RE, Friston KJ, Frackowiak RSJ: Regional cerebral blood flow during voluntary arm and hand movements in human subjects. J Neurophysiol 1991;65:1392–1401.

31 Ikeda A, Lüders HO, Burgess RC, Shibasaki H: Movement-related potentials recorded from supplementary motor area and primary motor area. Role of supplementary motor area in voluntary movements. Brain 1992; 115:1017–1043.

32 Aizawa H, Inase M, Mushiake H, Shima K, Tanji J: Reorganization of activity in the supplementary motor area associated with motor learning and functional recovery. Exp Brain Res 1991;84:668–671.

33 Luppino G, Matelli M, Rizzolatti G: Corticocortical connections of two electrophysiologically identified arm representations in the mesial agranular frontal cortex. Exp Brain Res 1990;82:214–218.

34 Luppino G, Matelli M, Camarda R, Rizzolatti G: Corticocortical connections of area F3 (SMA-proper) and area F6 (pre-SMA) in the macaque monkey. J Comp Neurol 1993;338:114–140.

35 Smith A, Bourbonnais D, Blanchette G: Interaction between forced grasping and a learned precision grip after ablation of the supplementary motor area. Brain Res 1981;222:395–400.

36 Roland PE, Larsen B, Lassen NA, Skinhoj E: Supplementary motor area and other cortical areas in organization of voluntary movements in man. J Neurophysiol 1980;43:118–136.

37 Shibasaki H, Sadato N, Lyshkow H, Yonekura Y, Honda M, Nagamine T, Suwazono S, Magata Y, Ikeda A, Miyazaki M, Fukuyama H, Asato R, Konishi J: Both primary motor cortex and supplementary motor area play an important role in complex finger movement. Brain 1993;116:1387–1398.

38 Jenkins IH, Brooks DJ, Nixon PD, Frackowiak RSJ, Passingham RE: Motor sequence learning: A study with positron emission tomography. J Neurosci 1994;14:3775–3790.

39 Tanji J, Shima K: Role for supplementary motor area cells in planning several movements ahead. Nature 1994; 371:413–416.

Dr. Eric M. Rouiller, Institut de Physiologie, Université de Fribourg,
Rue du Musée 5, CH–1700 Fribourg (Switzerland)

Hepp-Reymond M-C, Marini G (eds): Perspectives of Motor Behavior and Its Neural Basis.
Basel, Karger, 1997, pp 44–51

....

Balance Control during Movement: Why and How?[1]

Jean Massion

Laboratoire de Neurobiologie et Mouvements, CNRS, Marseille, France

In his illuminating paper, Hess [1] (see also Jung and Hassler [2]) explained why posture, equilibrium and movement need to be coordinated during the performance of most motor acts. He first explained that in standing humans, movements lead to both balance disturbance and postural destabilization. Balance disturbance results from the changes in the body's geometry due to the movement execution. For example, when an arm is raised forward by a standing subject, the arm's mass and center of inertia are shifted forward, and this would result in shifting the center of gravity (CG) forward and making it project onto the supporting surface closer to its anterior border. In addition, the internal muscular forces which are at the origin of the movement give rise to opposite reaction forces acting on the supporting segments such as the trunk, and consequently disturb the position of these segments. Prior to these two kinds of balance and postural disturbance, the planning of a given motor act includes not only controlling the movement of a segment toward a target, but also making 'anticipatory' postural adjustments so as to correct in advance the balance and postural disturbances due to the movement [3–6].

When a standing subject is performing forward arm raising movements, the internal muscular forces are directed forward and upward; the reaction forces due to the movement are transmitted to the trunk and are thus liable to cause the trunk position to shift backward and downward. The anticipatory postural adjustments associated with arm raising contribute to maintaining the initial trunk posture by initiating a trunk movement in a direction opposite to the reaction forces and thereby reducing the trunk displacement and the associated CG shift. Thus, the anticipatory postural adjustments which occur during arm raising serve a dual function: stabilizing the trunk position and greatly reducing the CG shift.

In other tasks, anticipatory postural adjustments have only one function. In a bimanual load lifting task, for example, the anticipatory postural adjustment of the 'postural' forearm serves to minimize the change in the forearm position resulting from the load lifting performed by the other arm [7, 8] and not, of course, to preserve balance. By contrast, when the upper trunk is moved forward or backward, the anticipatory postural adjustments serve only to preserve balance during the movement [9, 10]. Interestingly, the balance

[1] This work has been supported by the Centre National d'Etudes Spatiales (CNES).

control is achieved during these trunk movements by changing the positions of various body segments: the kinematic synergies first described by Babinski [11], characterized by movements of upper and lower segments in opposite directions, are the way in which balance is preserved during trunk movements.

The present paper will focus on the anticipatory control of balance during movement, in the hope of throwing some light on two important issues which are still a matter of controversy.

The first point concerns the variables controlled in equilibrium maintenance. What is actually controlled by the central nervous system (CNS) in order to preserve balance during quiet stance or during a voluntary movement: is it the body's geometry, the CG position with respect to the supporting base, or the ground reaction forces? The second question relates to the central organization of balance control during upper trunk movements: do two separate, parallel but coordinated controls exist, one dealing with balance and the other with the movement, or is there a single control which at the same time ensures that balance is maintained and that the movement is properly performed towards its goal?

Is the CG Position Controlled by the CNS?

In standing quadrupeds as well as in standing humans, under normal gravity conditions, balance control is mainly a force control task, which includes two aspects: producing the force level required to develop an erect posture against the gravity vector, and exerting the force in the appropriate direction to adapt the force vector to the support conditions and thus preserve balance [12].

Which variables are mainly controlled by the CNS when adjusting its reaction forces to the ground? It has been claimed by Lacquaniti [13] and by Fung and Macpherson [14] that the main value regulated in quadrupeds is the body's geometry, or more specifically, the orientation of body segments with respect to the external world, such as the verticality of the leg axis or the orientation of the trunk with respect to the ground. The actual CG position was thought to be not directly controlled, but to result from the geometrical configuration selected with respect to the external world. According to this theory, the control is therefore organized in terms of body geometry and not in terms of body mass.

The results of a series of investigations on humans which will be summarized here have argued against this idea, and suggest that it is the body mass, or more specifically the CG position in the horizontal plane which is directly controlled by the CNS [see 15].

A first interesting finding in this context was based on the fact that during fast trunk bending, which changes the body's geometry, other body segments are moved simultaneously in the opposite direction and as a result, the CG projection onto the ground remains within the supporting surface (fig. 1). As during fast movements the control is exerted in a feed-forward manner, it suggests that there exists an internal representation of the body segments' mass and inertia, which serves to coordinate the trunk movements with displacements of the lower segments in the opposite direction [9, 10].

Another finding was based on the effect of adding a load to the shoulders on the balance control during upper trunk movements [16]. When a 10-kg load is added to the shoulders of a standing subject it does not change the AP position of the CG with respect to the ground. When the subject is instructed to perform as fast as possible a trunk bending of the same amplitude as without load, the final CG position at the end of a trunk bending

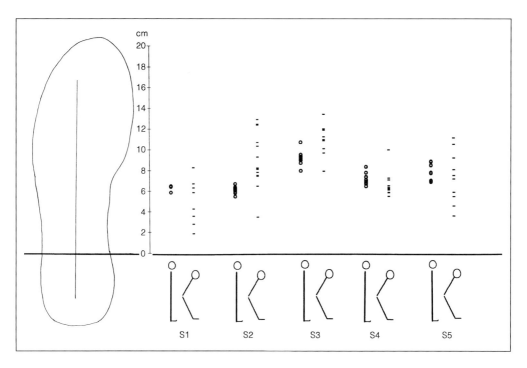

Fig. 1. Position of the CM before and 300 ms after the end of a forward trunk movement. The 5 subjects (S1, S2, S3, S4, S5) were instructed to perform the movement as fast as possible in response to a tone. On the left, the shape of the foot. On the right, the initial and final CM projection with each of the 5 subjects. Note that the initial position was located in a narrow zone in front of the ankle joint axis. At the end of the movement, the positions were more widely distributed but remained inside the support area.

movement would shift about 4 cm further forward or backward if the additional mass was not taken into account for the balance control during the movement. When the CG shift was measured with and without a load on the shoulders, it turned out that in 3 out of the 5 subjects, the final CG position remained the same whether or not the load was applied. In these subjects, the additional mass was taken into account by the system controlling the 'kinematic synergy' which minimized the final CG shift along the anteroposterior axis. This involved an internal representation of the additional mass, and a predictive evaluation of the CG shift to occur at the end of the movement. Finally, in microgravity, in absence of balance constraints, the center of mass (CM) shift with respect to the feet area is still minimized during upper trunk bending as in normogravity [see 17].

All in all, these findings argue in favor of the hypothesis that an internal representation of the body segments mass and inertia exists in addition to the representation of the body segments geometry [18]. This representation is used to adapt the distribution of the body segments in space in order to adjust the anteroposterior CG position with respect to the ground. However, as found to occur with arm raising [19], the balance constraints are an important factor involved in adjusting the CG position on the basis of this internal representation.

One should however bear in mind that during erect posture in normogravity, the balance (CM position with respect to the support surface) is not the only controlled variable during stance. A parallel control does exist, which specifies the body segments orientation with respect to the external world [15]. The 'load receptors' should play an important role in this orientation [20]. Examples are the vertical head axis orientation and the vertical trunk axis orientation which are maintained during stance and locomotion [21, 22]. In given tasks, changes in body segments configuration related to balance control are modifying the head or trunk axis with respect to vertical. This occurs, for example, during leg raising when the whole body is bending toward the supporting leg in order to shift the CG toward that leg. In order to preserve the head-trunk axis aline with vertical, a new coordinated control develops in dancers, by which a trunk movement around the hip joint compensates for the leg inclination around the ankle [23].

How is the CG Controlled during Movement?

During upper trunk bending, equilibrium control is a task which has to be carried out simultaneously with the movement execution. Generally speaking, when two goals have to be controlled simultaneously in a given motor task, two parallel controls take place in a coordinated way. During a reaching and grasping task, for example, two parallel controls seem to exist which are coordinated [24]. An alternative solution might arise after learning: the two goals may be achieved by a single control, in a similar way as it occurs during the learning of a single joint movement, where the dynamic disturbances occurring when the movement is executed are gradually cancelled by feed-forward adaptive networks which build up an appropriate inverse dynamic command [25]. A process of this kind might also be responsible for the organization of balance control during trunk movements. Another aspect of the control of trunk bending is worth mentioning here. During bending, opposite shifts of hip and knee are observed. The joints involved in the whole movement are the hip, the knee and the ankle, which correspond to 3 degrees of freedom (DF). In addition to the trunk bending there is an additional constraint, namely balance control. Two DF are needed for this dual task. There thus exists a redundancy in the number of DF. How the CNS deals with this redundancy is a question which still remains to be answered.

The kinematic, EMG and force platform data obtained in a study on upper trunk bending suggest that the CNS may use a single automatic control which simultaneously handles the movement velocity and amplitude on the one hand and stabilizes the CG position along the AP axis on the other, by fixing the ratio between the joint angle changes. The following items support the concept of a single automatic control:

(1) The EMG analysis showed that an early burst in the trunk, thigh and shank muscles preceded the movement onset. This finding indicates that the CNS exerts a simultaneous open loop command on the various segments which are involved in the kinematic synergy [9].

(2) The opposite movements of upper (shoulder) and lower segments (hip and knee) occur synchronously. The maximal peak velocity of the shoulder marker and that of the knee marker were time locked. If multijoint synergistic movements involved only dynamic interactions between segments, there would be a lag between the maximal velocity peaks of the various segments [26]. This suggests that the CNS probably takes part in the timing of synergies (fig. 2).

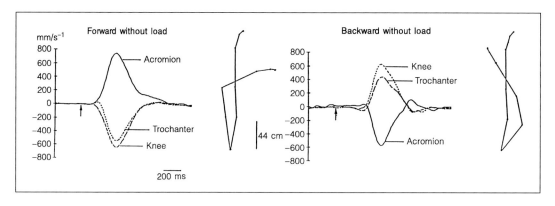

Fig. 2. Single trial recordings of the velocity curve of the acromion, trochanter and knee markers along the anteroposterior axis. The timing of the peak velocity of acromion, trochanter and knee markers remained synchronized in all the subjects during forward and backward trunk movements. The arrow indicates the tone signal onset. The stick diagrams give the initial and final positions of the segments during forward and backward upper trunk movements performed without additional load on the shoulder. The markers were located at the head (2 markers), acromion, trochanter, knee and ankle.

(3) A principal component analysis of the hip, knee, and ankle joint changes with respect to time was performed [27]. This mathematical analysis replaces the variations of the three angles involved in the task, the hip, knee and ankle joint by three principal components (PC1, PC2, PC3). Each PC represents a fixed ratio between the angle changes. If the movement is represented by only one principal component, then it means that a fixed ratio exists between the angle changes and that only 1 DF is controlled. The results accounted for that PC1 represented more than 99% of the total kinematic synergy in the case of forward movements and more than 96% in that of backward movements. This indicates that the kinematic synergy which occurs during upper trunk movement is similar to that involved in a 1 DF movement, with fixed ratios between the angle changes. As the same ratios are still observed between movements differing in their time courses, i.e., in their amplitude and velocity and hence in the interaction between segments, the 1 DF movement as reflected by PC1 does not result from only passive interactions between segments but from a central control system which organizes the kinematic synergy in terms of (a) the time course of the movement and (b) the ratios between the angle changes. Unlike PC1, PC2 was very weak and only present in fast movements. It probably reflects dynamic intersegmental disturbances which are not taken into account by the central control.

(4) In microgravity, the kinematic synergies involved in trunk bending are preserved, although the equilibrium constraints are absent or at least markedly reduced [28]. A similar situation has been found to occur under water, where the gravity vector is still present, but the equilibrium constraints associated with the body's weight are cancelled by the pressure of the water [29]. The data obtained in experiments carried out in microgravity and under water argue in favor of the hypothesis that the kinematic synergies are automatic motor patterns which serve to maintain the AP position of the CM during trunk movements, and that these memorized patterns persist even when the equilibrium constraints are absent.

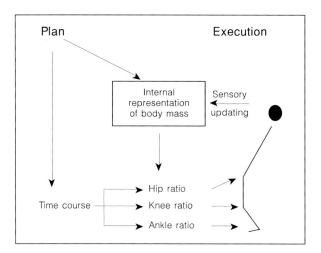

Fig. 3. Scheme indicating how balance is controlled during upper trunk movements. The control provides a time course signal and, on the base of an internal representation of the body mass and geometry, the fixed ratios between the angle changes. The internal representation may be updated by sensory signals informing on the balance constraints and the actual body mass.

Conclusions

The results of the above investigations, together with the data from the literature, indicate that the CM position along an anteroposterior axis is controlled during upper trunk movements, even in microgravity, where no balance constraints exist. They also show that the central control may adjust the CG position as a function of the actual mass when an external load has been added to the shoulders. Finally, the kinematic synergies which are responsible for the trunk movement and the CM stabilization are organized in the same way as a 1 DF movement.

In conclusion, the following general framework for the central organization of trunk bending movements is proposed in order to explain how balance is preserved during trunk movements (fig. 3).

(1) A memorized representation of the mass and inertia of the various segments seems to exist. This representation takes the form of an estimation of the position of each segment with respect to the vertical, and also includes an evaluation of its mass and inertia. On the basis of this internal representation, it is possible to estimate the forthcoming shift of the CG in the anteroposterior and lateral directions which will occur if a given segment is moved, and to determine which segment will have to be moved in the opposite direction in order to cancel this shift. For example, the angular shift of a segment such as the trunk by 30° with respect to the vertical will have to be accompanied by an angular shift of another segment, such as the shank, by 10° in the opposite direction, in order to preserve the same anteroposterior CG position. Therefore, a memorized representation of the angular ratios which maintain balance during movement seems to exist.

(2) This memorized representation of angular ratios which keeps the CG position steady on the AP or lateral axis may be updated when changes in given body segment

mass occur (at least when these changes of mass are among those which usually occur in every-day life). Any additional external load may be taken into account in the memorized angle ratios which are at the origin of the kinematic synergy.

(3) The memorized representation of angular ratios is not always used in an automatic fashion, but may be modified by a gain and gate control related to equilibrium constraints. In the case of upper trunk movements, the memorized representation of angular ratios is still operational in absence of equilibrium constraints, as for example in microgravity. This may be related to the fact that the trunk has the largest mass among the body segments, and that trunk movements are the main source of balance disturbance during daily life. In contrast, with arm movements which disturb much less balance, the kinematic synergies which reduce the CG shift during the movement are weak during bipedal stance. However, when the balance constraints are increased, such as during unipedal stance, the CG shift is minimized, and the kinematic synergies increased.

(4) The simultaneous control of movement velocity and amplitude and that of the CG position is achieved quite simply. This control has two main aspects. The first one is the time course signal, which defines the movement amplitude and velocity. The second aspect is the ratio between the angle changes. A fairly simple control system of this kind can be compared to the concept of the generalized motor program proposed by Schmidt [30]. How a simple kinematic control system such as that responsible for kinematic synergies may be transformed to deal with the torque control of individual angles is still a matter of speculation. The equilibrium point theory extended to multijoint control might be a basis for this kind of control, as proposed by Feldman and Levin [31].

References

1   Hess W: Teleokinetisches und ereismatisches Kräftesystem in der Biomotorik. Helv Physiol Pharmacol Acta 1943;1:C62–C63.
2   Jung R, Hassler R: The extrapyramidal motor system; in Field J, Magoun HW, Hall VE (eds): Handbook of Physiology, sect 1, Neurophysiology, vol 2, chap 35. Bethesda, American Physiological Society, 1960.
3   Belenkii VE, Gurfinkel VS, Paltsev EI: On elements of control of voluntary movements (in Russian). Biofizica 1967;12:125–141.
4   Bouisset S, Zattara M: Biomechanical study of the programming of anticipatory postural adjustments associated with voluntary movement. J Biomech 1987;20:735–742.
5   Cordo PJ, Nashner LM: Properties of postural adjustments associated with rapid arm movements. J Neurophysiol 1982;47:287–302.
6   Massion J: Movement, posture and equilibrium: Interaction and coordination. Prog Neurobiol 1992;38:35–56.
7   Hugon M, Massion J, Wiesendanger M: Anticipatory postural changes induced by active unloading and comparison with passive unloading in man. Pflügers Arch 1982;393:292–296.
8   Kaluzny P, Wiesendanger M: Feedforward postural stabilization in a distal bimanual unloading task. Exp Brain Res 1992;92:173–182.
9   Crenna P, Frigo C, Massion J, Pedotti A: Forward and backward axial synergies in man. Exp Brain Res 1987;65:8–548.
10   Oddsson L, Thorstensson A: Fast voluntary trunk flexion movements in standing motor patterns. Acta Physiol Scand 1987;129:93–106.
11   Babinski J: De la synergie cérébelleuse. Rev Neurol (Paris) 1899;17:806–816.
12   Macpherson JM, Deliagina TG, Orlovsky GN: Control of body orientation and equilibrium in vertebrates; in Stein PSG, Grillner S, Selverston AI, Stuart DG (eds): Neurons, Networks, and Motor Behavior. Cambridge/Mass, MIT Press, 1996.
13   Lacquaniti F: Automatic control of limb movement and posture. Curr Opin Neurobiol 1992;2:807–814.
14   Fung J, Macpherson J: Determinants of postural orientation in quadrupedal stance. J Neurosci 1995;15:1121–1131.
15   Massion J: Postural control system. Curr Opin Neurobiol 1994;4:877–887.
16   Vernazza S, Alexandrov A, Massion J: Is the center of gravity controlled during upper trunk movements? Neurosci Lett 1996;206:77–80.

17   Massion J, Mouchnino L, Vernazza S: Do equilibrium constraints determine the center of mass position during movement? In Mergner T, Hlavacka H (eds): Multisensory Control of Posture. New York, Plenum Press, 1995, pp 103–107.

18   Clément G, Gurfinkel VS, Lestienne F, Lipshits MI, Popov KE: Adaptation of postural control to weightlessness. Exp Brain Res 1984;57:61–72.

19   Vernazza S, Cincera M, Pedotti A, Massion J: Balance control during lateral arm raising in humans. Neuroreport 1996;206:77–80.

20   Dietz V: Neuronal basis of stance regulation. Interlimb coordination and antigravity receptor function; in Swinnen SP, Heuer H, Massion J, Casaer P (eds): Interlimb Coordination: Neural, Dynamical, and Cognitive Constraints. New York, Academic Press, 1994, pp 167–178.

21   Berthoz A, Pozzo T: Intermittent head stabilization during postural and locomotory tasks in humans; in Amblard B, Berthoz A, Clarac F (eds): Posture and Gait: Development, Adaptation and Modulation. Amsterdam, Elsevier, 1988, pp 189–198.

22   Assaiante C, Amblard B: Ontogenesis of head stabilization in space during locomotion in children: Influence of visual cues. Exp Brain Res 1993;93:499–515.

23   Mouchnino L, Aurenty R, Massion J, Pedotti A: Coordination between equilibrium and head-trunk orientation during leg movement: A new strategy built up by training. J Neurophysiol 1992;67:1587–1598.

24   Jeannerod M: The Neural and Behavioral Organization of Goal-Directed Movements. Oxford, Clarendon Press, 1988.

25   Ito M: A new physiological concept of cerebellum. Rev Neurol 1990;146:564–569.

26   Ramos CF, Stark LW: Simulation experiments can shed light on the functional aspects of postural adjustments related to voluntary movements; in Winters JM, Woo L-Y (eds): Multiple Muscle Systems: Biomechanics and Movement Organization. New York, Springer, 1990, pp 507–517.

27   Alexandrov A, Frolov A, Massion J: Principal component analysis of axial synergies during upper trunk forward bending in human; in Mergner T, Hlavacka F (eds): Multisensory Control of Posture. New York, Plenum Press, 1995, pp 95–101.

28   Massion J, Gurfinkel V, Lipshits M, Obadia A, Popov K: Axial synergies under microgravity conditions. J Vestib Res 1993;3:275–287.

29   Massion J, Fabre J-C, Mouchnino L, Obadia A: Body orientation and regulation of the center of gravity during movement under water. J Vestib Res 1995;5:211–221.

30   Schmidt RA: Motor Control and Learning. A Behavioral Emphasis, ed 2. Champaign/Ill, Human Kinetic Publishers, 1988.

31   Feldman AG, Levin MF: The origin and use of positional frames of reference in motor control. Behav Brain Sci 1995;18:723–806.

Dr. Jean Massion, Laboratoire de Neurobiologie et Mouvements, CNRS,
31, chemin Joseph Aiguier, F–13402 Marseille Cedex 20 (France)

Hepp-Reymond M-C, Marini G (eds): Perspectives of Motor Behavior and Its Neural Basis.
Basel, Karger, 1997, pp 52–56

....
Quantitative Analysis of Complex Movements

Antonio Pedotti

Centro di Bioingegneria, Fondazione Don Gnocchi IRCCS–Politecnico di Milano, Italy

Studies on motor control in humans have been focused mainly on reflex responses and simple voluntary movements involving one or two joints, with the rest of the body being usually constrained or neglected. On the other hand, many neurophysiological studies have investigated various stereotyped performances executed by invertebrates or lower animals.

Therefore, very few comprehensive quantitative data on motor tasks executed in everyday life are present in the literature, even if it clearly appears that motor control mainly relies on the concept of goal-oriented movements which require a global coordination. Such a process has to take into account different problems, including coordination of multiple limbs in three dimensions, maintenance of dynamic equilibrium, sharing of muscle forces and loads on various body segments, and a predetermined level of accuracy, speed, mechanical power, etc. These essential features which allow us to associate motor organization to the more general concept of intelligence have often been underestimated.

Etienne-Jules Marey and Edward Muybridge, towards the end of the last century, were the first able to document the complexity of motor performance with the introduction of photographic movement analysis. Their beautiful pictures showed the coordination between the various parts of the body, but they were not suitable to provide detailed quantitative data which require a precise analysis in the three-dimensional (3D) space.

It is only in recent years that analyses have included more complex movements, often involving the whole body, performed by 'freely behaving', unconstrained subjects. One of the main reasons for this new trend is certainly the availability of improved technologies, which make it possible to collect and process data in a more rapid and reliable way, with minimal interference on the subject's performance [1]. Another reason is most probably the necessity to avoid or minimize the artifactual aspects of the experimental condition by dealing with voluntary movements as much as possible within the natural repertoire of everyday life. Indeed, in such movements a distinctive feature of the motor system is maximally exploited, namely the possibility to execute a same motor task through different combinations of muscle forces and/or kinematics (i.e. with different strategies). Such an operational redundancy, which implies a peculiar organization of the control mechanisms, exceeding the classical concepts of control theory, will optimally adapt the resulting movement to the specific individual and environmental demand.

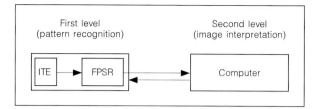

Fig. 1. Architecture of the ELITE system.

The analysis of these aspects, as well as the identification of the various strategies adopted in complex movements, requires a rigorous investigation of different kinds of variables including kinematics, forces and EMG. Starting from these data, suitable mathematical models are available for the computation of other parameters which cannot be measured directly (e.g. mechanical moments acting at the joints, muscle lengths, etc.). The new technologies combined with the modelling approach provide a powerful tool to investigate with great accuracy complex movements.

After a brief description of the optoelectronic systems for movement analysis, I will present investigations which are possible by these 'magnification lenses'. The analysis of interindividual variability in human gait shows that different individuals are using different motor strategies and that all these different strategies minimize the total muscular effort in line with an invariant goal achievement with variable means.

Automatic Movement Analysis

The recent developments in image-processing techniques (pattern recognition, computer vision, etc.) and in parallel computation by fast VLSI chips allowed in the mid-80s the development of a new generation of fully automatic systems for the automatic 3D analysis of movement. The ELITE system [1] performs the data collection in several steps that are hierarchically organized and share some features with the visual systems of human beings [2–4]. First, the body segments, the movement of which is to be analyzed, are recognized. This reduces the complexity of the scenery into a few relevant primitives. Second, the two-dimensional (2D) coordinates of these primitives are computed and the distortions introduced by the surveying system are also corrected. In order to achieve a 3D analysis, more than one sensor is used and additional steps are required: these are the matching of the same primitives in different images and the computation of 3D coordinates. The innovative feature of the ELITE system is the marker detection hardware which works on the shape and size of the markers rather than on their brightness. This characteristic allows a very easy use of the system even in sunlight. The architecture of the system is hierarchically organized in two levels (fig. 1). The lower or first level is represented by the interface to the environment (ITE) and by the fast processor for shape recognition (FPSR): the higher or second level is implemented on a commercial personal computer. The ITE includes markers of different dimensions according to the field of view. They range from 0.8 mm to 15 mm depending on the field of view. This flexibility allows the system to be used for very different set-ups. The lighting system is realized by a circular ring of IRLEDSs coaxial with the lenses, strobed in order to obtain sharp pictures without come-tail effect. The TC cameras adopted are of the solid-state CCD type which allow the best definition in the images at a sampling frequency of 50 or 100 Hz. In addition, an electronic internal shutter system contributes to increase the signal-to-noise ratio and allows the recognition of the markers in the daylight. The second block of the first level is the FPSR. This constitutes the core of the system and performs the recognition of the markers and the computation of their coordinates. Its implementation has been done by using fast VLSI chips in a pipe-lined structure. This first level sends to the computer the 2D coordinates of the markers as registered during the movement. The second level is software implemented on a traditional serial personal computer and it performs high-level processing [5]: image interpretation, dealing with marker classification, 2D calibration, 3D intersection and further processing such as filtering, computing derivatives, modelling, etc. Between the first and second level a further step is carried out. By using a coordinate enhancement algorithm, taking into account the cross-correlation function, the resolution is increased to 1/65,000 of the field of view [1].

Individual Strategies in Normal Gait

In a study of normal gait [6] in a group of young male subjects walking on a walkway at a natural speed, EMGs from the main lower limb muscles, kinematics and ground reactions were recorded. The EMG patterns of all subjects are within the normal 'range of variability' usually reported for human gait (fig. 2). But, when they are individually correlated with the other biomechanical variables these patterns show a consistent interindividual variability (fig. 2). This concerns particularly the interplay between the biarticular hamstrings (extensors at hip and flexor at knee) and the monoarticular vasti (extensors at knee).

In subject A, the activity of hamstrings starts immediately before the heel strike, increases immediately thereafter and lasts up to the middle of the stance phase (ST). In contrast, in subjects B and C, the hamstring activity reaches its maximum at or before the heel strike, and stops immediately thereafter. The vasti are slightly activated in subject A while displaying an increasing level of activity in subject B which is particularly strong and long-lasting during ST in subject C. In this last subject a bimodal activity of the calf muscles which is not present in subjects A and B can also be observed.

A question arises at this point: Can these differences in amplitude and timing of EMG patterns be associated with other independent variables so that they can be reasonably interpreted as a component of a more complex individual motor strategy? The comparison with the time course of moments computed independently from kinetics and ground reaction measurements confirms that the different EMG patterns are the part of a well-defined and intraindividually variable dynamic behavior. In fact, in subject A a hip extensor and knee flexor moment pattern starts at the end of swing phase and lasts for almost the entire stance. In both cases, these moments are supported by the long-lasting activity of the hamstrings, with the second part of the flexor moment at the knee being supported by the calf muscles.

In subject B and especially in C, the knee extensor moment is significatively higher and therefore the hamstrings stop their activity immediately after the onset of the stance, in conjunction with a more pronounced activity of vasti. Also, the bimodal time course of moment at the ankle is associated with the bimodal calf activity in subject C.

This close matching between individual EMG patterns and mechanical variables, observed in each subject, excludes that interindividual differences in amplitude and timing

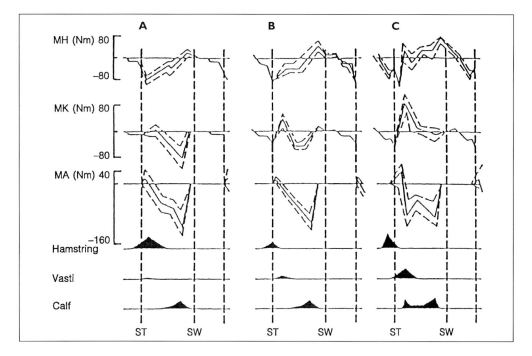

Fig. 2. Multifactorial analysis of a gait cycle in 3 subjects: (**A–C**). On the abscissa the normalized time is reported, divided in stance phase (ST) and swing phase (SW). On each column from top to bottom are reported the mechanical moments active on the plane of progression at hip (MH), knee, (MK), and ankle (MA) joint, respectively. The positive values represent a flexor action at the hip, an extensor action at the knee and a dorsal flexion at the ankle. Mean values of the moments and the range of uncertainty are illustrated by the continuous and dashed lines, respectively. For sake of simplicity, the activity of the main muscles has been grouped in hamstrings, including biceps femoris, semitendinosus and semimembranosus, vasti and calf including soleus and gastrocnemius. EMG envelopes are a schematization of the integral, filtered activity, normalized with respect to the maximal voluntary contraction.

of muscles activities could be attributed to random variability around a basic pattern, suggesting the existence of different individual motor strategies. A previous study [7] has shown that these individual patterns in level walking are consistent with a minimization of the total muscle effort.

Conclusions

Other investigations of complex voluntary movements, like axial movements [8, 9], lifting a leg [10], jumping from a platform [11], have been recently performed by using the 'magnification lenses', the optoelectronic systems for 3D movement analysis. These studies demonstrate the existence of well-defined individual patterns of muscle recruitment associated with biomechanical variables during the execution of the same performance under the same experimental conditions. In several groups of subjects, like high-level athletes or dancers, the individual motor programs are clearly aimed at optimizing performance. Whether or not such programs are the result of learning or are genetically transmitted remains an open question. However, the results show that in complex movements the achievement of the goal is an invariance, that the means are variable and the overall performance is optimized thanks to the intrinsic redundancy of the motor system.

References

1   Ferrigno G, Pedotti A: ELITE: A digital dedicated hardware system for movement analysis via real-time TV signal processing. IEEE Trans Biomed Eng 1985;32:943–950.
2   Ullman S: The Interpretation of Visual Motion. Cambridge/Mass, MIT Press, 1979.
3   Marr D, Vaina L: Representation and recognition of the movements of shapes. Proc R Soc Lond [B], 1982; 214:501–524.
4   Poggio GF, Poggio T: The analysis of stereopsis. Annu Rev Neurosci 1984;7:379–412.
5   Ferrigno G, Borghese NA, Pedotti A: Pattern recognition in 3D automatic human motion analysis. ISPRS J Photogr Remote Sens 1990;45:227–246.
6   Pedotti A, Crenna P: Individual strategies of muscle recruitment in complex natural movements; in Winters JM, Woo SL-Y (eds): Multiple Muscle Systems: Biomechanics and Movement Organization. New York, Springer, 1990, pp 542–549.
7   Pedotti A, Krishnan VV, Stark L: Optimization of muscle-force sequencing in human locomotion. Math Biosci 1978;38:57–76.
8   Crenna P, Frigo C, Massion J, Pedotti A: Forward and backward axial synergies in man. Exp Brain Res 1987; 65:538–548.
9   Pedotti A, Crenna P, Deat A, Frigo C, Massion J: Postural synergies in axial movements: Short- and long-term adaptation. Exp Brain Res 1989;74:3–10.
10 Mouchnino L, Aurenty R, Massion J, Pedotti A: Coordination between equilibrium and head-trunk orientation during leg movement: A new strategy built up by training. J Neurophysiol 1992;67:1587–1598.
11 McKinley P, Pedotti A: Motor strategies in landing from a jump: The role of skill in task execution. Exp Brain Res 1992;90:427–440.

Dr. Antonio Pedotti, Centro di Bioingegneria, Fondazione Don Gnocchi IRCCS–Politecnico di Milano, Via Capecelatro 66, I-20148 Milan (Italy)

Hepp-Reymond M-C, Marini G (eds): Perspectives of Motor Behavior and Its Neural Basis.
Basel, Karger, 1997, pp 57–64

....

Locomotor Training in Paraplegic Patients

Volker Dietz [1]

Swiss Paraplegic Centre, University Hospital Balgrist, Zürich, Switzerland

For more than 30 years, functional electrical stimulation of paralyzed limb muscles represented the sole approach to improve the mobility of paraplegic patients [1]. Despite some technical developments, this method is still in its experimental stage and no breakthrough leading to a more extensive application has been achieved [2]. This is mainly due to basic problems such as rapid development of muscle fatigue and adverse interactions with spinal reflexes which can hardly be solved by technical means. During recent years a new approach which overcomes these shortcomings has been established. This approach consists of an external activation and training of spinal locomotor centers. This review highlights some of the recent developments in this field which may be of some benefit for improving the motor function and mobility in incomplete paraplegic patients.

Physiological Background

The recovery of locomotor function after a spinal cord transsection in cat was believed for several years to be restricted to an immature stage [3]. Later on, it could be demonstrated that the recovery of the locomotor pattern can be considerably improved by regular training, even in the adult cat [4]. During this locomotor training, the animal was supported and had only to bear a part of its body weight. Locomotor movements of the hindlimbs were induced by a moving treadmill while the forelimbs stood on a platform. With ongoing training, body support was decreased according to the cat's locomotor abilities. After some weeks of training, the cat was able to completely take over its body weight during well-coordinated stepping movements [5]. The locomotor pattern at this stage closely resembled the pattern of intact adult cat [6]. Thus it could be concluded that the training represents an important factor for the recovery of locomotor function.

In human, step-like movements are present at birth and can be initiated spontaneously or by peripheral stimuli. The electromyographic (EMG) activity underlying this newborn stepping has been shown to be centrally programmed and, as it has also been observed

[1] I thank Dr. Gibson for advice on presentation. This work was supported by the Swiss National Science Foundation (No. 31–42899.95) and the International Research Institute for Paraplegia (P16/93).

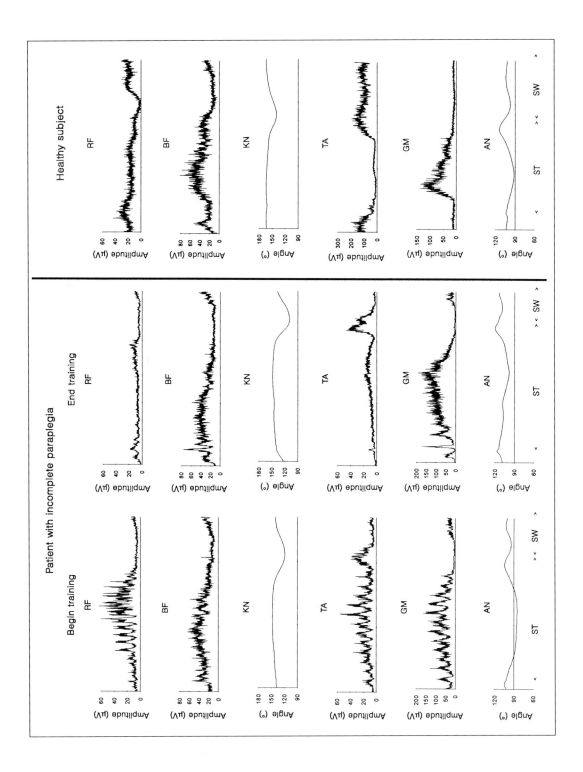

in anencephalic children, it is likely that spinal mechanisms generate the EMG activity [7]. The apparent loss of locomotor movements in accidentally spinalized humans has been suggested to be due to a greater predominance of supraspinal over spinal neuronal mechanisms [8]. Nevertheless, there are some indications in humans that spinal interneuronal circuits exist which are involved in the generation of locomotor EMG activity in the leg muscles (for review, see Dietz [9], similar to those described for the cat [6]). Furthermore, involuntary stepping-like leg movements were recently described in a subject with a neurologically incomplete injury to the cervical spinal cord [10].

Effect of Locomotor Training in Paraplegic Patients

The aim of several recent studies was to evaluate the degree to which locomotor EMG activity and movements can be both elicited and trained in leg muscles of both complete and incomplete paraplegic patients [11–15].

The induction of complex bilateral leg muscle activation combined with coordinated stepping movements in incomplete and complete paraplegics was achieved by partially unloading (up to 60%) the body weight of patients who were on a moving treadmill. The leg movements had to be assisted by external persons during the first phases of the training in the incomplete patients (fig. 1). The assistance lasted during the whole training period (3–5 months) in all complete paraplegic patients (fig. 2). In comparison to healthy subjects, the paraplegic patients displayed a less dynamic mode of muscle activation. This may be due to the impaired function of polysynaptic and monosynaptic spinal reflexes in patients with a spinal lesion [16]. In other respects, such as the timing, the pattern of leg muscle EMG activity was similar to that recorded in healthy subjects. Different EMG-amplitude levels in the leg extensor (the main antigravity muscle during gait) occurred in the different subject groups and they largely exceeded the normal inter-individual variability [17]. The amplitude level of EMG activity was considerably smaller in complete as compared to incomplete paraplegics, and in the latter group compared to healthy subjects. Despite the reduced EMG activity, spastic symptoms (e.g. increased muscle tone, exaggerated reflexes) were present in both patient groups. This supports earlier notions claiming that alterations of the mechanical muscle fiber properties in the tonically active muscle are mainly responsible for the clinical signs of spasticity [16, 18, 19; for review, see 9].

One may argue that the EMG pattern observed during the locomotor training in complete paraplegic patients may be due to rhythmic stretches of the leg muscles. From the ankle joint recordings displayed in figures 1 and 2 and from figure 3 it becomes obvious that the EMG activity in leg muscles is about equally distributed between muscle lengthening and shortening in healthy subjects and patients during locomotion. This indicates that

Fig. 1. Rectified and averaged (n = 20) EMG activity of lower and upper leg muscles together with knee and ankle joint movements during slow locomotion (around 1.3 km/h) in a healthy subject (right) and an incomplete paraplegic patients (left). For the patient the recordings at the beginning and after a daily performed locomotor training over 5 months are displayed. The amount of unloading for the healthy subject was 40 of 80 kg; for the patient, see figure 4. At the end of training the EMG amplitude of the GM muscle is larger and less clonus-like. In addition, there is less TA coactivation during the ST phase. The EMG activation in GM has a longer duration during ST in the patient than in the healthy subject. RF = Rectus femoris; BF = biceps femoris; KN = knee joint; TA = tibialis anterior; GM = gastrocnemius medialis; AN = ankle joint; ST = stance; SW = swing phase. From Dietz et al. [15].

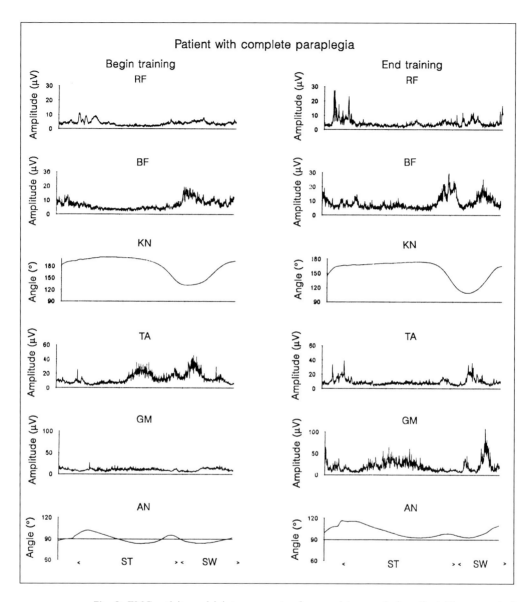

Fig. 2. EMG activity and joint movements of a complete paraplegic patient. The amount of unloading is indicated in figure 4. At the end of training the EMG activity of the GM muscle had increased in amplitude, but was still considerably smaller than in the healthy subject and incomplete paraplegic patient displayed in figure 1. Therefore, the locomotor movements had to be assisted (see text; from Dietz et al. [15].) For details and abbreviations, see figure 1.

stretch reflexes are unlikely to play a major role in the generation of the leg muscle EMG pattern, but that they are rather programmed at a spinal level.

During the course of a daily locomotor training program, the amplitude of gastrocnemius EMG activity increased significantly during the stance phase, while an inappropriate tibialis anterior activation decreased. These training effects were seen in both groups,

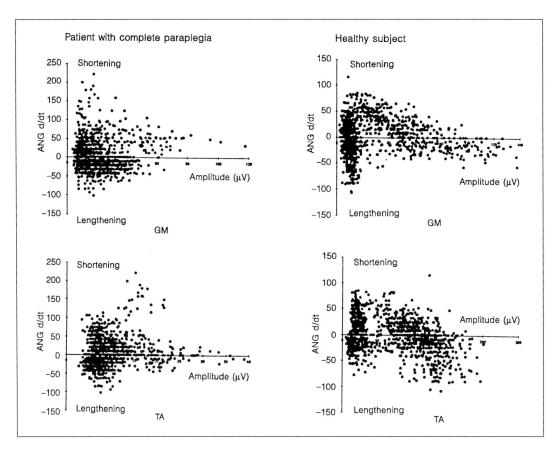

Fig. 3. Relationship between muscle lengthening and shortening (velocity at the ankle, ANG d/dt, °/s) and EMG amplitude in the gastrocnemius medialis (GM, top) and tibialis anterior (TA, bottom) within a step cycle (EMG amplitude measured every 100 ms). Left: complete paraplegic patient. Right: healthy subject. There is an almost equal distribution of EMG amplitude during muscle lengthening and shortening for both GM and TA muscles.

incomplete and complete paraplegic patients (fig. 4). This was related to the greater weight-bearing function of the extensors. The slope of increase was similar in incomplete and complete paraplegics. This indicates that the isolated human spinal cord contains the capacity not only to generate a locomotor pattern, but also 'to learn'. The latter finding is an agreement with a recent observation made in healthy subjects [20, 21]. Nevertheless, apart from positive effects upon the cardiovascular and musculoskeletal systems, only incomplete paraplegic patients benefitted from the training program with respect to the performance of unsupported stepping movements on solid ground [14, 15]. In contrast to leg extensor, only a small training effect on the leg flexor EMG amplitude was seen. This may be due to a differential neuronal control of leg flexor and extensor muscles during locomotion [22]. The progressive reloading of the body during training may serve as a stimulus for extensor load receptors which have been shown to be essential for the leg extensor activation during locomotion in cat [23] and man [24]. It is assumed that the load receptor information arises from Golgi tendon organs and is mediated by group Ib

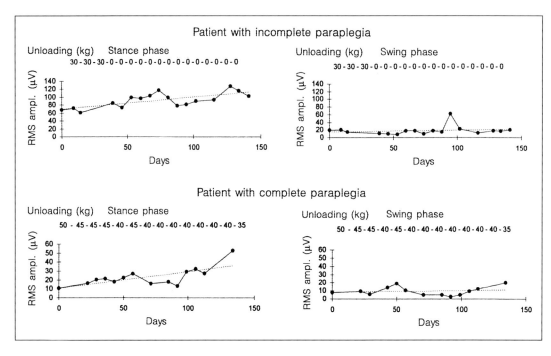

Fig. 4. Quantified gastrocnemius EMG during the stance (left) and swing (right) phases for an incomplete (left) and a complete (right) paraplegic patient (same patients as in figures 1 and 2 respectively). Each point represents the mean value of one recording session (usually weekly). The slope of increase in gastrocnemius EMG activity during stance within the training period was significant for both patients ($r = 0.7$, $p < 0.005$). The amount of body weight unloading is indicated above the upper and lower diagrams. The activity level on the ordinate is expressed as root mean square (RMS). There is a nearly linear increase in EMG amplitude during the training period in both the incomplete and complete paraplegic patient. This increase takes place, however, on a higher EMG background level in the incomplete paraplegic patient. From Dietz et al. [15].

afferents to the spinal locomotor centers [23]. The lower gain of extensor EMG in complete paraplegic patients may be due to a loss of input from descending noradrenergic pathways to spinal locomotor centers [5].

Pharmacological Influences on Locomotor Activity

In a recent study, no training effect was seen in about half of patients with complete paraplegia [15]. The *a posteriori* analysis led to the suggestion that this might be due to the action of the drugs taken by the patients. Cannabinoids [25] and Prazosin (an α_1-adrenoceptor antagonist) [6] are drugs which are known to inhibit spinal neuronal activity. In contrast to this, it had been previously demonstrated that the administration of clonidine enhances locomotor activity in spinal cats [26]. Nevertheless, a contrary effect was seen in 2 patients after intrathecal application of a low dose (25 µg) of clonidine (fig. 5). This was connected with a loss of EMG activity and with flaccid paresis [15]. While a species-dependent action seems rather unlikely for this observation, there may be several explana-

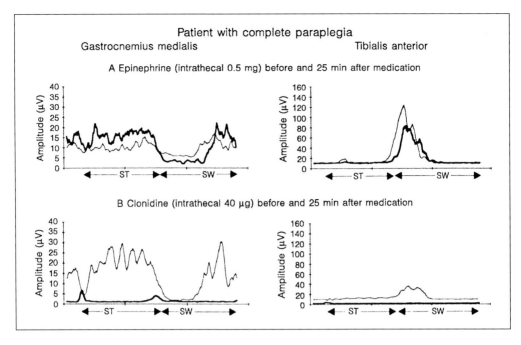

Fig. 5. Rectified and averaged (n = 20) gastrocnemius (left) and tibialis anterior (right) EMG activity of a complete paraplegic patient before (thin lines) and after (heavy lines) intrathecal application of epinephrine (**A**) and clonidine (**B**). While the application of epinephrine results in moderate increase in the gastrocnemius EMG activity during ST, clonidine causes a dramatic drop in EMG amplitude associated with flaccid muscle tone. From Dietz et al. [15]. For details and abbreviations, see figure 1.

tions for the differential effect seen between cat and man, for example, a dosage- or 'level of lesion'-dependent change of the drug action. In contrast to clonidine, the sympathomimetic drug epinephrine was shown to have a positive effect on the locomotor pattern and performance (fig. 5). This suggests that human spinal locomotor activity can be influenced by pharmacological means. Further studies are required to determine the degree to which human spinal locomotor activity can be positively influenced by other (nor-) adrenergic agonists, thereby supporting the locomotor training. Furthermore, detailed and controlled investigations are needed, particularly bearing in mind that significant neuronal changes may occur in untreated patients during the first months following spinal cord injury.

Conclusion

In conclusion, recent studies on paraplegic patients have shown that, similar to the cat, a spinal locomotor pattern generator also exists in man. In paraplegic patients, a locomotor pattern can be induced and can be trained. However, at present, only incomplete paraplegic patients profit from this training for their locomotor abilities. In addition to the training effects, pharmacological treatment can also influence the locomotion pattern. Both training and pharmacology represent new approaches to improve the mobility of paraplegic patients.

References

1   Kantrowitz A: Electronic Physiologic Aids. Brooklyn, NY. Report of the Maimonides Hospital, 1960, pp 4–5.
2   Quintern J, Minwegen P, Mauritz K-H: Control mechanisms for restoring posture and movements in paraplegics;
    in Allum JHJ, Hulliger M (eds): Afferent Control of Posture and Locomotion. Prog Brain Res. Amsterdam,
    Elsevier, 1989, vol 80, pp 489–502.
3   Forssberg H, Grillner S, Halbertsma J, Rossignol S: The locomotion of the low spinal cat. II. Interlimb
    coordination. Acta Physiol Scand 1980;108:283–295.
4   Barbeau H, Rossignol S: Recovery of locomotion after chronic spinalization in the adult cat. Brain Res 1987;
    412:84–95.
5   Barbeau H, Rossignol S: Enhancement of locomotor recovery following spinal cord injury. Curr Opin Neurol
    1994;7:517–524.
6   Grillner S: Control of locomotion in bipeds, tetrapods, and fish; in Brookhart M, Mountcastle VB (eds):
    Handbook of Physiology. The Nervous System, vol II, Motor Control, part 2. Washington, American Physiologi-
    cal Society, 1981, pp 1179–1236.
7   Forssberg H: A developmental model of human locomotion; in Grillner S, Stein PSG, Stuart DG, Forssberg
    H, Herman RM (eds): Wenner-Gren International Symposium Series. Neurobiology of Vertebrate Locomotion
    London, Macmillan, 1986, vol 45, pp 485–501.
8   Kuhn RA: Functional capacity of the isolated human spinal cord. Brain 1950;73:1–51.
9   Dietz V: Human neuronal control of automatic functional movements. Interaction between central programs
    and afferent input. Physiol Rev 1992;73:33–69.
10 Calcanie B, Needhom-Shropshine B, Jacobs P, Willer K, Zych G, Breen BA: Involuntarily stepping after chronic
    spinal cord injury: Evidence for a central rhythm generator for locomotion in man. Brain 1994, 117:1143–1199.
11 Visintin M, Barbeau H: The effects of body weight support on the locomotor pattern of spastic paretic patients.
    Can J Neurol Sci 1989;16:315–325.
12 Barbeau H, Fung J: New experimental approaches in the treatment of spastic gait disorders; in Forssberg H,
    Hirschfeld H (eds): Movement Disorders in Children. Med Sport Sci. Basel, Karger, 1992, vol 36, pp 234–246.
13 Wernig A, Müller S: Laufband locomotion with body weight support improved walking in persons with severe
    spinal cord injuries. Paraplegia 1992;30:229–238.
14 Dietz V, Colombo G, Jensen L: Locomotor activity in spinal man. Lancet 1994;344:1260–1263.
15 Dietz V, Colombo G, Jensen L, Baumgartner L: Locomotor capacity of spinal cord in paraplegic patients. Ann
    Neurol 1995;37:574–582.
16 Dietz V, Quintern J, Berger W: Electrophysiological studies of gait in spasticity and rigidity: Evidence that
    altered mechanical properties of muscle contribute to hypertonia. Brain 1981;104:431–449.
17 Horstmann GA, Gollhofer A, Dietz V: Reproducibility and adaptation of the EMG responses of the lower leg
    following perturbations of upright stance. Electroencephalogr Clin Neurophysiol 1988;70:447–452.
18 Ibrahim IK, Berger W, Trippel M, Dietz V: Stretch-induced electromyographic activity and torque in spastic
    elbow muscles. Differential modulation of reflex activity in passive and active motor tasks. Brain 1993;116:
    971–989.
19 Sinkjaer T, Toft E, Larsen K, Andreassen S, Hansen H: Non-reflex and reflex mediated ankle joint stiffness in
    multiple sclerosis patients with spasticity. Muscle Nerve 1993;16:69–76.
20 Gordon CR, Fletcher WA, Melvill Jones G, Block EW: Adaptive plasticity in the control of locomotor trajectory.
    Exp Brain Res 1995;102:540–545.
21 Prokop T, Berger W, Zijlstra W, Dietz V: Adaptational and learning processes during split-belt locomotion:
    Interaction between central mechanisms and afferent input. Exp Brain Res 1995;106:449–456.
22 Dietz V, Horstmann GA, Berger W: Interlimb coordination of leg-muscle activation during perturbation of
    stance in humans. J Neurophysiol 1989;62:680–693.
23 Pearson KG, Collins DF: Reversal of the influence of group Ib afferents from plantaris on activity in medial
    gastrocnemius muscle during locomotor activity. J Neurophysiol 1993;70:1009–1017.
24 Dietz V, Gollhofer A, Kleiber M, Trippel M: Regulation of bipedal stance: Dependency on 'load' receptors.
    Exp Brain Res 1992;89:229–231.
25 Meinck HM, Schönle PW, Conrad B: Effect of cannabinoids on spasticity and ataxia in multiple sclerosis. J
    Neurol 1989;236:120–122.
26 Barbeau HJ, Julien C, Rossignol S: The effects of clonidine and yohimbine on locomotion and cutaneous
    reflexes in the adult chronic spinal cat. Brain Res 1987;437:83–96.

Dr. Volker Dietz, Swiss Paraplegic Centre, University Hospital Balgrist,
Forchstrasse 340, CH–8008 Zürich (Switzerland)

Hepp-Reymond M-C, Marini G (eds): Perspectives of Motor Behavior and Its Neural Basis.
Basel, Karger, 1997, pp 65–76

....

Motor Phenomena during Sleep

Gabriella Marini [1]

Istituto di Neuroscienze e Bioimmagini, Consiglio Nazionale delle Ricerche, Milano, Italy

This chapter is concerned with motor activity in sleep. First, an analysis of physiological motor events occurring during sleep is attempted. The second part of the chapter deals with certain parasomnias (sleep disorders), which are characterized by particular motor phenomena that may provide clues to the biological basis of disturbances in human motor control. Finally, some own findings on the effects of restricted thalamic lesion experiments in cats are summarized, focusing on electromyographic (EMG) recordings that help in understanding the mechanisms of myoclonic jerks in sleep.

Normal Motor Phenomena of Sleep

For the sake of brevity, only bodily shifts, cortical excitability, the atonia of rapid eye movement (REM) sleep, reflexes, hypnic physiologic myoclonias, and myoclonic jerks will be discussed. No attempt will be made to review the large body of literature concerning eye movements.

Bodily Shifts

In the 19th century, the newly available photographic techniques that were used to depict animal and human motion in sequences [1] were not applied to the study of sleep. This was probably because sleep was erroneously considered to be an inert and largely motionless state. At that time, it was also assumed that the brain shut off in sleep. Ninety years later, Theodore Spagna's time-lapse photographic studies [2] documented that, although spontaneous or responsive movements are reduced, even the soundest sleepers shift position at least 8 times during the night.

Human sleep is characterized by episodes of immobility punctuated by major postural shifts. The organization of this motor activity was shown to be periodic and related to the electroencephalographic (EEG) sleep cycle, i.e. the period of alternation of synchronized and desynchronized sleep (or paradoxical or REM sleep) phases. Major body movements occur mainly in transition from non-REM (NREM) to REM sleep and again when REM gives away to the next NREM phase, but not during either the progression of the 4 stages of the synchronized NREM or fully established REM sleep. These movements involve

[1] I am grateful to Profs A. Hobson, P. Montagna, and M. Wiesendanger who provided useful comments on a previous version of this paper.

slow changes in the position of the whole body or of limbs so that the same position is not maintained for too long a time, thus preventing paralysis onset due to prolonged compression of some peripheral nerves, even if transient and reversible. In fact, everyone has experienced waking up with sensations of 'pins and needles' (night acroparesthesia), numbness and hampered in movements. In general, the phenomenon disappears in a few minutes, but chronic alcoholics who fall deeply asleep after overdrinking and lie resting immobile with their heads on their forearms for a prolonged period of time, may sustain paralysis of the radial nerve, the so-called 'Saturday evening paralysis' that takes up to a few days or weeks to recede.

Cortical Excitability

The changes in motor activity occurring during the sleep cycle have raised the question whether cortical excitability was also modified during different behavioral states. With the advent of techniques for recording discharges of single neurons in unanesthetized and unrestrained animals, it was possible to study patterns of neuronal activity during natural sleep and waking. Evarts [3] showed that the discharge pattern of pyramidal tract cells rather than their overall activity changed during sleep in monkeys. These neurons which regularly discharged during waking, exhibited bursts and periods of silence during slow wave sleep, and displayed increase of the length of bursts and intervening periods of silence during REM sleep (fig. 1). Evarts thought that this change in pattern might be due to a progressive loss of inhibition. In fact, he reported that motor cortical neurons that remained unidentified antidromically (presumed interneurons) has lower rates of spontaneous firing and in the majority exhibited changes across the sleep-waking cycle opposite to that of the pyramidal tract cells. In subsequent studies [4], cortical interneurons have been recorded in the monkey motor cortex and cat parietal association areas and identified electrophysiologically. It was confirmed that cortical interneurons decreased their discharge rate or stopped firing on arousal and progressively increased their discharge rate as the animal falls asleep.

The availability of a method to stimulate the human motor cortex painlessly through the intact scalp (transcranial magnetic stimulation, see Hess et al., chap. 9) has permitted the re-investigation of the excitability of central motor structures during sleep. It could then be demonstrated that the response of the human motor cortex to stimulation is depressed during NREM sleep and enhanced during REM sleep (fig. 2) [5].

Atonia of REM Sleep

REM sleep is defined by a trilogy of cardinal physiological correlates: EEG desynchronization, rapid eye movements and EMG suppression. The apparently paradoxical presence of REM sleep atonia coupled with a high level of activity of central neurons (including those of motor systems) is the most striking motor phenomenon occurring during sleep. Although the function of this behavioral state remains unclear, the mechanisms that control the lack of antigravity tone during REM sleep are now well understood.

Jouvet et al. [6] first described the complete relaxation of postural muscles during paradoxical sleep. Measuring the electric activity of neck muscles, Jouvet et al. found that the transition from the EEG synchronization of NREM sleep to the EEG desynchronization of REM sleep was associated with electrical silence in antigravity muscles. Extracellular and reflex studies (see below) [for review, see 7] indicated that muscle atonia is the consequence of tonic postsynaptic inhibition of spinal ventral horn neurons by the pontomedullary reticular formation. The discharges of two groups of neurons, one in the anterodorsal pontine tegmentum (monaminergic neurons of the peri-locus coeruleus α) and one in the medullary

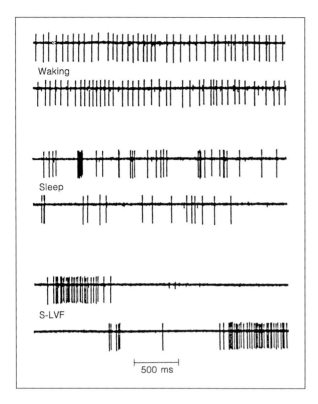

Fig. 1. Modification in discharge pattern of pyramidal tract neurons occurring during waking, sleep, and sleep with low-voltage fast EEG activity (S-LVF, i.e. REM) in the monkey. During waking discharge tends to be regular; during sleep there are bursts interspersed with periods of relative inactivity; during S-LVF burst duration increases and periods of inactivity become longer. From Evarts [3], with permission.

reticular formation (magnocellular nucleus) are strongly correlated with muscle tone obliteration [8]. This association has fostered the hypothesis of a pontomedullary-spinal circuit with the pontine neurons being excitatory to medullary elements which, in turn, are inhibitory to the ventral horn neurons. Intracellular recordings of medial bulbar reticular formation neurons in naturally sleeping cats indicate the presence of a REM-specific tonic membrane depolarization that occurs close to the onset of muscle atonia and lasts throughout the REM state and thus support the hypothesis [9].

Reflexes

The striking collapse of antigravitary tone occurring during REM sleep has led several investigators to analyze the problem of the modulation of spinal reflexes during waking and sleeping in more detail. Reflex excitability is slightly depressed during the NREM sleep phase, but significant changes occur during REM sleep. In man, it has been observed that H-reflex is depressed during REM sleep [10]. In cat, it was found that the heteronymous monosynaptic reflex and the polysynaptic flexion reflex which greatly fluctuate during attentive waking, become more stable during light sleep and tend to be abolished during

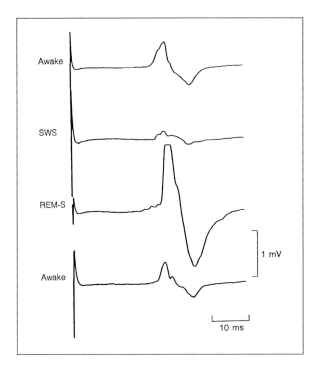

Fig. 2. Compound muscle action potential recorded with surface electrodes from right abductor digiti minimi in response to magnetic stimuli applied at the vertex during the waking state, slow wave sleep (SWS), REM sleep and the waking state again. The response in REM sleep is more than twice as large as that in the waking state. The stimulus was given during an actual REM episode. From Hess et al. [5], with permission.

REM sleep [11–13]. Spinal cord section studies indicated that such abolition was due to descending inhibitory volleys impinging upon the reflex arcs during REM sleep [14–16]. Further studies showed that two different types of inhibitory processes were acting during this state, a tonic one lasting through the whole REM episode and a phasic one accompanying the rapid eye movements and muscles twitches especially of distal flexor muscles. A series of investigations provided the evidence that the phasic inhibition was of presynaptic nature: during REM sleep the positive component of the cord dorsum potential evoked by electrical stimulation of group I afferents was reduced (fig. 3) [14], the antidromic spike amplitude of dorsal roots was increased (due to primary afferent depolarization of terminals of Ia fibers) [15], and slow waves spontaneously appeared in the electrospinogram (fig. 4) [16]. These findings strongly suggest that increased presynaptic inhibition (induced by supraspinal structures) causes the reflex depression. The postsynaptic origin of the tonic inhibition was at a later stage demonstrated by intracellular recordings from antidromically identified lumbar motoneurons in naturally sleeping cats [17, 18]. The presence of a marked hyperpolarization of motoneuronal membrane coincident with the loss of neck EMG activity suggest that increased inhibition is the basis of the REM sleep atonia [18].

Evidence is accumulating that muscle atonia of REM sleep may involve more than one anatomically and pharmacologically specific brainstem system. It is noteworthy that reflex depression and atonia during REM sleep are accompanied by the suppression of

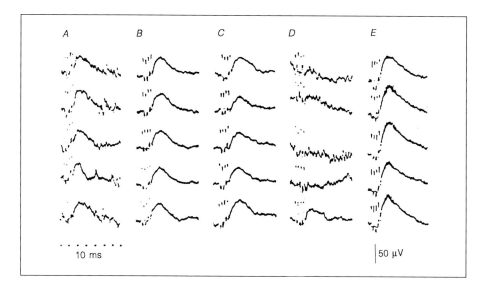

Fig. 3. Cord dorsum potentials evoked by a train of 4 impulses (applied at 300 Hz, 0.02 ms duration) to posterior biceps semitendinosous group I fibers. The positive component (P wave) reaching a maximum after 20–25 ms from the first stimulus, appeared to be rather stable and present for every train of stimuli during relaxed wakefulness (**A**) and did not change consistently as the animal passed from waking to synchronized sleep (**B**). During REM sleep no tonic variation of the cord dorsal potential was ever observed (**C**). Instead, the P wave appeared phasically reduced and often disappeared synchronously with the spontaneous electrospinogram slow waves which were generally present at the same time as the periods of the most intense REMs of desynchronized sleep (**D**). The P wave of cord dorsum potential markedly increased both in amplitude and duration after the intravenous injection of an anesthetic dose of pentobarbital (**E**). From Baldissera et al. [15], with permission.

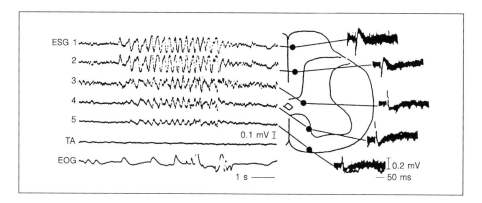

Fig. 4. Electrospinographic slow wave activity synchronous with a REM episode as seen in the EOG and TA activity (on the left) and field potentials evoked by four Ia stimuli to deep peroneal nerve recorded at various depths within the lumbar enlargement (on the right). Note positivity of the first deflection of the spinal slow waves and of the field potential when recorded from points 1 and 2 and reversal in polarity of both when derived from electrodes 3, 4 and 5. No muscular twitch is present in anterior tibial (TA) myogram. From Baldissera and Broggi [16] with permission.

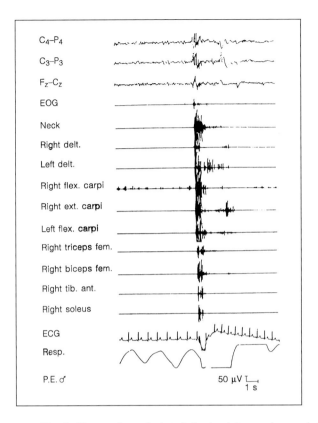

C₄–P₄	
C₃–P₃	
Fz–Cz	
EOG	
Neck	
Right delt.	
Left delt.	
Right flex. carpi	
Right ext. carpi	
Left flex. carpi	
Right triceps fem.	
Right biceps fem.	
Right tib. ant.	
Right soleus	
ECG	
Resp.	
P.E. ♂	50 µV / 1 s

Fig. 5. Nocturnal myoclonic twitches involving synchronously the trunk and limb muscles. Note that the violent muscular contractions involve all the body muscles including the respiratory ones. From Coccagna [23], with permission.

spontaneous activity of locus coeruleus and raphe neurons. The findings are in accord with the concept that these state-dependent tonic excitability changes of spinal motor mechanisms may be mediated by the noradrenergic [19, 20] in addition to the cholinergic system, proposed by Pompeiano [7].

Hypnic Physiologic Myoclonias and Myoclonic Jerks

Hypnic physiologic jerks consist of brief, jerky contractions of a muscle or groups of muscles and are normal in the course of falling asleep and during REM sleep. De Lisi [21] first described the partial myoclonias as rapid, asymmetric, and asynergic muscular contractions which involve a restricted portion of the muscle inducing small movements. Face and distal limb muscles are mainly affected. Myoclonic twitches are rapid and there are strong contractions of the trunk and limb muscles. Oswald [22] described the sudden bodily jerks on falling asleep as axial movements associated with the K-complex, a biphasic EEG wave followed by a high-voltage slow wave. Figure 5 illustrates the violent muscular contractions which involve simultaneously all body muscles including the respiratory ones. They are often associated with hallucinoid imagery, autonomic storms (flurries of heart and respiratory rates, sweating) and are followed by awakening or by a lighter sleep [23].

Motor Disorders Arising during Sleep

Significant progress in the understanding of sleep disorders has been made in specialized sleep laboratories with all-night video and polysomnographic studies (recordings of EEG, EMG, EOG and other vegetative parameters).

Parasomnias are defined as episodic dysfunctions in sleep that intrude into the sleep process but do not primarily cause complaints of insomnia. They involve either the motor system or the respiratory system or the cognitive system. I will concentrate on the parasomnias characterized by motor disturbances of sleep, in particular: sleepwalking, REM-sleep behavior disorder, restless legs syndrome, nocturnal paroxysmal dystonia, and bruxism. These phenomena consist in a release of patterned motor activities which seem inappropriate for sleep. They may provide clues for understanding disturbances of human motor activity.

Sleepwalking

> Doctor to Lady Macbeth:
> 'A great perturbation in nature, to receive at once
> The benefit of sleep, and do the effects of watching!'
> W. Shakespeare, Macbeth, Act V, Sc. I

Sleepwalking, so poetically described by Shakespeare, is one of the major motor disorders during sleep. This dysfunction occurs in NREM sleep and without accompanying mental activity [24]. In fact, if awakened, the patient is not able to report any organized mental activity. Typical episodes last for about 10 min, and during this time the individual may demonstrate complex behavior. The high prevalence of these disorders in children prior to puberty and their resolution after puberty suggests that sleepwalking may be related to central nervous system maturation factors [25].

REM-Sleep Behavior Disorder (RBD)

RBD is a recently described condition. A wide range of motor behavior – some fragmentary, some elaborate – occurs in association with REM sleep [26]. When waking up, the RBD patients often remember a dream, the content of which fits with the observed motor behavior. All events of REM sleep (EEG activation, ocular movements) occur except the atonia. In fact, in EMG recordings, tonic activity is present. This abnormal motor disinhibition during REM sleep was anticipated by earlier animal experiments. Following lesions in the anterodorsal pons [27], sequences of automatic movements were seen in cats in conjunction with all the other EEG signs of REM sleep. This was especially true when the lesions disconnected the upper pons from the lower brainstem [28]. Such lesions are thought to have interrupted the pathway of the peri-locus coeruleus neurons, which project to and excite the medullary inhibitory reticular formation cells and thus inhibit the spinal motoneurons. Jouvet and Delorme [27] suggested that these movements were a rehearsal of elementary motor behaviors. In humans, the RBD is typically observed in patients who often develop degenerative disorders of the central nervous system such as dementia, Parkinson's disease, and olivopontocerebellar atrophy several years after the first RBD attacks.

Restless Legs Syndrome (RLS)

The clinical description of RLS dates back to the 17th century, but Ekbom [29] gave the first detailed description of the clinical features. Despite intensive investigation, many physiopathological and therapeutic questions remain largely unsolved. The syndrome is

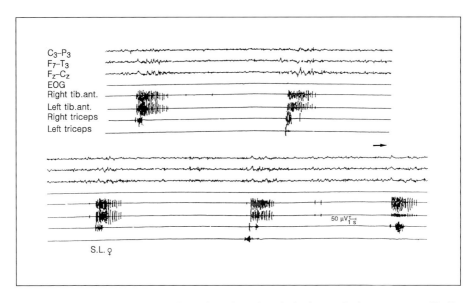

Fig. 6. RLS: polysomnographic tracings show that rhythmic myoclonias occur every 35–40 s during light sleep. In this case, they involve both limbs, but predominate in tibialis anterior muscles. From Coccagna [23], with permission.

characterized by the occurrence of uncomfortable and difficult to define sensations, in the legs between the knee and the ankle. They begin in the evening while the patient is at rest, are exacerbated when subjects lie in bed and fall asleep. RLS is almost always accompanied by nocturnal myoclonus [30], now defined as periodic movements in sleep. Figure 6 shows the rhythmic myoclonia occurring every 35–40 s and affecting the anterior tibialis muscles of both limbs. RLS in sleep in normal subjects are closely linked to age: virtually absent in subjects under 30, they reach a peak incidence of 29% over age 50. In RLS, the unpleasant sensations induce an irresistible need to move the legs, and often oblige the patient to get up and walk. Movement may reduce the paresthesic sensations, but they reappear as soon as the patient lies down. Sometimes, due to the high frequency of their occurrence, they may prevent sleep. Rarely, the symptoms affect the arms. RLS may be found in association with chronic myelopathies and neuropathies and other diseases such as chronic respiratory insufficiency. Family studies are suggestive of an autosomal dominant mode of inheritance [31].

Nocturnal Paroxysmal Dystonia (NPD)

NPD is a new type of motor disorder related to NREM sleep, recently identified by means of polysomnographic studies [32]. NPD consists of strong, vigorous movements occurring often with dystonic or dyskinetic components. The patient opens his eyes, raises or turns his head to one side and assumes a dystonic posture that usually involves head, trunk, and all four limbs. In addition, he may display wide, violent, and stereotyped dyskinetic movements, such as jerky flexion-extension of the trunk, ballistic movements of the upper or lower limbs or violent torsional movements around the body axis. The motor attack is associated with generalized EEG desynchronization. NPD was previously considered a parasomnia. Recently the epileptic nature of these episodes has been established. The epileptic focus resides in the frontal mesial regions (frontal lobe nocturnal epilepsy). The syndrome may occur as an autosomal dominant trait linked to a mutation in the α-subunit of the neuronal nicotinic ACh receptor [33].

Bruxism

Bruxism (tooth grinding) is a type of abnormal craniocervical and orofacial movements that occur during sleep. It manifests itself as clenching and rhythmic, jerky muscle activity. In addition to the series of brief rhythmic contractions of the masticatory muscle, hypertrophy or pain of masseter and temporal muscles are observed [34]. Patients with bruxism have been shown to have little disruption of nocturnal sleep. Several physiopathological mechanisms have been proposed to explain bruxism. Local factors such as tooth interference, hyperactivity of the dopaminergic system, and emotional stress may be etiological factors.

Evidence for the Involvement of the Posterior Intralaminar Thalamus in Myoclonias as Revealed by Excitotoxic Injections in Cats

The role of the medial thalamus in the regulation of sleep, emphasized by Hess [35], was challenged, and the hypothalamus and reticular formation favored as sleep-regulating centers. Recently, a case report of fatal familial insomnia [36] with severe neuronal thalamic degeneration has renewed the importance of the thalamus in the regulation of sleep.

We have investigated the effects of bilateral ibotenic acid microinjections in various thalamic nuclei on the electrographic correlates of sleep. When the target was the posterior intralaminar centre médian (CM) [37], the immediate (therefore excitatory) effect was a highly aroused behavior associated with cortical activation, eye movements, pontogeniculo-occipital waves, and prominent muscle tone (fig. 7A), suggesting orienting-like behavior. Spontaneous, stereotyped twitches began in the neck muscles and forelimbs, and were fully developed 2–3 h postinjection. Quasi-periodic discharges of motor units were recorded from the neck muscles which often occurred in doublets and triplets (fig. 7B). Repetitive myoclonic jerks occurred every 5–10 s during waking, but their frequency decreased to one per 10–20 s when the EEG became synchronized (fig. 7C), and disappeared in deeper sleep stages when the EEG became fully synchronized. Sometimes the jerk occurred at the transition from NREM to waking (fig. 7D), closely resembling the hypnic jerks described in man. These jerks were never associated with paroxysmal EEG activity suggestive of epilepsy. The overaroused behavior fits with the traditional role conferred to the thalamic intralaminar complex which is considered to mediate the reticular activation of the cortical EEG that characterizes both waking and REM sleep states. In the light of the hodology of the posterior intralaminar group, many various roles have been ascribed to CM. Based on human neuropathological material [38] and on lesion experiments in the monkey [39], it has been suggested that the thalamic CM nucleus plays a central role in the mechanisms of certain dyskinesias and particularly, in the genesis of myoclonic jerks. The privileged links with the striatal structures, which are known to be involved in experimental myoclonus [40], may mediate the effects induced in forelimbs and neck muscles by the excitotoxin. Such myoclonias have some resemblance to human partial hypnic myoclonias, suggesting a common physiological mechanism.

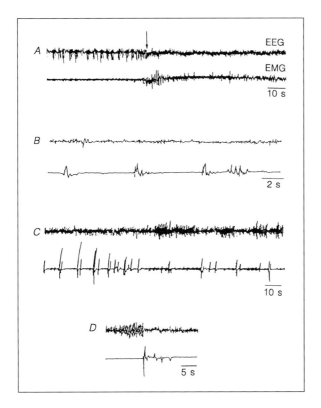

Fig. 7. Effect of ibotenic acid injections into the CM thalamic nucleus on EMG activity in the cat. **A** Immediately after the injection (arrow), prominent muscle tone associated with EEG desynchronization. **B** 2–3 h postinjection, spontaneous, sterotyped twitches recorded in neck muscles. **C** Sustained myoclonic jerks occurring every 5–10 s during waking and decreasing in frequency and amplitude when the EEG became synchronized. **D** Example of jerk occurring at the transition from NREM to waking, closely resembling the hypnic jerks described in man. Modified from Mancia and Marini [37].

Conclusion

From this brief review it is apparent that the various sleep cycles have profound effects on the motor system. Learning more about the motor manifestations during sleep may help us to understand the physiological and pathological mechanisms associated with various sleep stages. Investigations of patients with sleep disorders will inspire parallel and well-controlled experiments in animals. Such an interdisciplinary effort should provide a mutual enrichment in the field of motor behavior and neurobiology of state control. Noninvasive brain imaging techniques coupled with the electro- and magneto-encephalography, will provide the tools to study the structures controlling not only the transition from sleep to an alert state, but also the transition from relaxed wakefulness to high levels of attention.

References

1   Muybridge E: Animal Locomotion: An Electro-Photographic Investigation of Consecutive Phases of Animal Movements. Dover Pictorial Archive Series. Mineola/NY, Dover Publications, 1887.

2   Hobson JA, Spagna T, Malenka R: Ethology of sleep studied with time-lapse photography: Postural immobility and sleep-cycle phase in humans. Science 1978;201:1251–1253.

3   Evarts EV: Temporal patterns of discharges of pyramidal tract neurons during sleep and waking in the monkey. J Neurophysiol 1964;27:152–171.

4   Steriade M: Cortical long-axoned cells and putative interneurons during the sleep-waking cycle (with commentaries). Behav Brain Sci 1978;3:465–514.

5   Hess CW, Mills KR, Murray NMF, Schriefer TN: Excitability of the human motor cortex is enhanced during REM sleep. Neurosci Lett 1987;82:47–52.

6   Jouvet M, Michel F, Courjon J: Sur un stade d'activité electrique cerebrale rapide au cours du sommeil physiologique. C R Soc Biol (Paris) 1959;153:1024–1028.

7   Pompeiano O: The neurophysiological mechanisms of the postural and motor events during desynchronized sleep. Proc Assoc Res Nerv Ment Dis 1967;45:352–423.

8   Sakai K, Sastre J-P, Kanamori N, Jouvet M: State-specific neurons in the ponto-medullary reticular formation with special reference to the postural atonia during paradoxical sleep in the cat; in Pompeiano O, Ajmone Marsan C (eds): Brain Mechanism and Perceptual Awareness. New York, Raven Press, 1981, pp 405–429.

9   Chase MH, Enomoto S, Murakami R, Nakamura Y, Taira M: Intracellular potential of medullary reticular neurons during sleep and wakefulness. Exp Neurol 1981;71:226–233.

10   Hodes R, Dement WC: Depression of electrically induced reflexes (H-reflexes) in man during low voltage EEG 'sleep'. EEG Clin Neurophysiol 1964;17:617–629.

11   Giaquinto S, Pompeiano O, Somogyi I: Supraspinal modulation of heteronymous monosynaptic and polysynaptic reflexes during natural sleep and wakefulness. Arch Ital Biol 1964;102:245–281.

12   Giaquinto S, Pompeiano O, Somogyi I: Descending inhibitory influences on spinal reflexes during natural sleep. Arch Ital Biol 1964;102:282–307.

13   Baldissera F, Broggi G, Mancia M: Spinal reflexes in normal unrestrained cats during sleep and wakefulness. Experientia 1964;20:1–3.

14   Gassel MM, Marchiafava PL, Pompeiano O: An analysis of the supraspinal influences acting on motoneurons during sleep in the unrestrained cat. Modifications of the recurrent discharge of the alpha motoneurons during sleep. Arch Ital Biol 1965;103:25–44.

15   Baldissera F, Cesa-Bianchi MG, Mancia M: Phasic events indicating presynaptic inhibition of primary afferents to the spinal cord during desynchronized sleep. J Neurophysiol 1966;29:871–887.

16   Baldissera F, Broggi G: An analysis of potential changes in the spinal cord during desynchronized sleep. Brain Res 1967;6:706–715.

17   Morales F, Chase MH: Intracellular recording of lumbar motoneuron membrane potential during sleep and wakefulness. Exp Neurol 1978;62:821–827.

18   Morales F, Chase MH: Postsynaptic control of lumbar motoneuron excitability during active sleep in chronic cat. Brain Res 1981;225:279–295.

19   Fung SJ, Barnes CD: Locus coeruleus control of spinal cord activity; in Barnes CD (ed): Brainstem Control of Spinal Cord Function. New York, Academic Press, 1984, pp 215–255.

20   Palmeri A, Wiesendanger M: Concomitant depression of locus coeruleus neurons and of flexor reflexes by an α_2-adrenergic agonist in rats: A possible mechanism for an alpha-2-mediated muscle relaxation. Neuroscience 1990;34:177–187.

21   De Lisi L: Su di un fenomeno motorio costante del sonno normale: Le mioclonie ipniche fisiologiche. Riv Patol Nerv 1932;29:481–496.

22   Oswald I: Sudden bodily jerks on falling asleep. Brain 1959;82:92–103.

23   Coccagna G: Il sonno e i suoi disturbi. Progressi Clinici: Medicina, Padova, Piccin, 1992, vol 6.

24   Kales A, Kales JD: Recent findings in the diagnosis and treatment of disturbed sleep. N Engl J Med 1974;290;487–499.

25   Kales A, Soldatos CR, Caldwell AB, et al: Sleepwaking, Arch Gen Psychiatry 1980;37:1406–1410.

26   Schenck CH, Bundlie SR, Ettinger MG, Mahowald MW: Chronic behavioral disorders of human REM sleep: A new category of parasomnia. Sleep 1986;9:293–308.

27   Jouvet M, Delorme JF: Locus coeruleus et sommeil paradoxal. C R Soc Biol (Paris) 1965;159:895–899.

28   Henley K, Morrison AR: A re-evaluation of the effects of lesions of the pontine tegmentum and locus coeruleus on phenomena of paradoxical sleep in the cat. Acta Neurobiol Exp 1974;34:215–232.

29   Ekbom KA: Restless legs syndrome. Neurology 1960;10:868–873.

30   Lugaresi E, Cirignotta F, Coccagna G, Montagna P: Nocturnal myoclonus and restless legs syndrome; in Fahn S, Marsden CD, Van Woert M (eds): Advances in Neurology, vol 43: Myoclonus. New York, Raven Press, 1986, pp 295–307.

31   Montagna P, Coccagna G, Cirignotta F, Lugaresi E: Familial restless legs syndrome: Long-term follow-up; in Guilleminault C, Lugaresi E (eds): Sleep/Wake Disorders: Natural History, Epidemiology, and Long-Term Evolution. New York, Raven Press, 1983, pp 231–235.

32   Lugaresi E, Cirignotta F, Montagna P: Nocturnal paroxysmal dystonia. J Neurol Neurosurg Psychiatry 1986; 49:375–380.
33   Steinlein OK, Mulley JC, Propping P, Wallace RH, Phillips HA, Sutherland GR, Sheffer IE, Berkovic SF: A missense mutation in the neuronal nicotinic acetylcholine receptor alpha-4-subunit is associated with autosomal dominant nocturnal frontal lobe epilepsy. Nat Genet 1995;11:201–203.
34   Velly-Miguel AM, Montplaisir J, Rompré PH, Lund JP, Lavigné JB: Bruxism and other oro-facial movements during sleep. J Craniomandib Disord 1992;6:71–81.
35   Hess WR: The sleep syndrome as elicited by diencephalic stimulation; in Akert K (ed): Biological Order and Brain Organization. New York, Springer, 1981, pp 131–169.
36   Lugaresi E, Medori R, Montagna P, Baruzzi A, Cortelli P, Lugaresi A, Tinuper P, Zucconi M, Gambetti P: Fatal familial insomnia and dysautonomia with selective degeneration of thalamic nuclei. N Engl J Med 1986; 315:997–1003.
37   Mancia M, Marini G: Orienting-like reaction after ibotenic acid injections into the thalamic centre médian nucleus in the cat. Arch Ital Biol 1995;134:65–80.
38   Schulman S: Bilateral symmetrical degeneration of the thalamus: A clinico-pathological study. J Neuropathol Exp Neurol 1957;16:446–470.
39   Milhorat TH: Experimental myoclonus of thalamic origin. Arch Neural 1967;17:365–378.
40   Patel S, Slater P: Analysis of the brain regions involved in myoclonus produced by intracerebral picrotoxin. Neuroscience 1987;20:687–693.

Dr. Gabriella Marini, Istituto di Neuroscience e Bioimmagini, CNR,
Via Fratelli Cervi 93, I–20090 Segrate-Milano (Italy)

Hepp-Reymond M-C, Marini G (eds): Perspectives of Motor Behavior and Its Neural Basis.
Basel, Karger, 1997, pp 77–90

....

Slow Cortical Potentials Developing Prior to a Self-Paced Voluntary Movement and in a Forewarned Reaction Time Task

A Study in Epileptic Patients with Implanted Electrodes

P. Buser, M. Lamarche, J. Louvel

Centre de Neurophysiologie clinique et Département de Neurochirurgie,
Hôpital Ste Anne, Paris, France

Electroencephalographic studies with scalp recording in normal subjects have amply described and documented a variety of slow potentials in relation to situations in which the subject was asked to perform a movement (arm, hand, leg or foot). Two distinct protocols were widely used. The first was a complex paradigm, with two separate stimuli, a *warning stimulus* to which the subject was instructed not to move, followed after 2–3 s by a second, *the imperative stimulus*, to which the subject had to execute a given movement. Most often, the warning stimulus was a light flash or a tone burst and the imperative stimulus, a series of flashes or tones that the subject had to interrupt through button press. The most conspicuous electrical phenomenon occurring with this paradigm was the well-known contingent negative variation (CNV), a slow scalp negative potential with large distribution, starting soon after the first stimulus and increasing until application of the second one. Initially described by Walter et al. [1], this 'expectancy' wave was then thoroughly studied by others [see e.g. 2–4]. Some of those (especially Brunia [3]) preferred to consider the CNV paradigm as that of a 'forewarned reaction time task'. In most cases the CNV itself started after the evoked potential to the warning stimulus and terminated at delivery of the imperative stimulus, which itself elicited a second evoked potential with several components.

A second set of scalp slow potentials accompanying movement was described by Kornhuber and Deecke [5] as 'Bereitschaftspotentiale', or 'readiness potential' (RP) and then studied by several groups [6–10]. It is a slow negative variation which precedes the performance of a voluntary self-paced movement (e.g. flexion of a finger, flexion of the forearm, the subject being instructed to perform it at irregular intervals). Just like the CNVs, the RP is widely distributed over the scalp with, however, some dominance on the side opposite to the moving body part. It comprises several components, the RP itself starting about 1,500 ms before the movement and then replaced after about 1,000 ms, i.e. 500 ms before the movement, by another component with a steeper slope, called 'negative shift' (NS). During the movement itself, a third, fast positive component is visible (premotor positivity, PMP), followed by a 'motor potential', before returning to the baseline.

Comparisons between the two types of event-related potentials were undertaken by several groups who particularly analyzed the content of the CNV. The CNV protocol is in fact a very complex one, and as precisely pointed out by several authors, involves at least two distinct mental processes: the attentive expectation for the second stimulus and the preparation to move. This latter process might thus be similar to that of a subject preparing to perform a self-paced movement [for discussions, see 11–14].

Having mainly in mind the localization of the generators responsible for the two types of slow potentials, we were fortunate to be able to perform recordings from epileptic patients who were under exploration with electrodes implanted for therapeutic purposes (localization of their epileptic focus). On this occasion a variety of issues could be raised regarding these potentials, their shape, their spatial distribution and their mutual relationships [15, 16].

Methods

So far, 35 patients suffering from drug-resistant partial epileptic seizures were investigated. Some of them had no permanent neurological deficits while others suffered from a hemisyndrome (hemiparesis or hemiplegia). None of them showed any major overt cognitive deficit while performing in our tests or in daily interactions. They were all under reduced antiepileptic therapy (sodium valproate, hydantoin, barbiturates, carbamazepine, vigabatrin, depending on the patient's symptomatology).

To localize their epileptic focus, the patients were implanted with chronic, multilead depth electrodes introduced into sites corresponding to the clinical and electroclinical characteristics of their seizures. Three to 7 days after implantation, they underwent several sessions of stereoelectroencephalographic (SEEG) recording of their ongoing activity, as well as a variety of electrical stimulations, to provide information on the localization of their epileptic focus. They usually had from 5 to 10 implanted electrodes. Each electrode had a diameter of 0.8 mm, and had either 5, 10 or most frequently 15 leads (each stainless steel lead being 2 mm long with a recording surface of 5 mm^2 and 2 successive leads being 1.3 mm apart). These electrodes were placed according to Talairach's stereotaxic coordinate system [17, 18]. Details on the methodology can be found in Rektor et al. [15] and Lamarche et al. [16]. Since the objective of the depth explorations was to delimit the epileptic focus in each case, the electrode placements were determined on the basis of the clinical and EEG information gathered during preliminary examination of the patient. These placements involved a variety of cortical areas of the convexity: premotor cortex, rolandic motor or sensory cortices, posterior parietal cortex, temporal cortex (superior, middle or inferior) and, on the mesial aspect of the hemispheres, the supplementary motor and the cingulate areas (anterior, middle and posterior), and more deeply the temporo-limbic structures such as amygdala, hippocampus or hippocampal gyrus. The only levels that were not explored in our series were the frontal and the occipital poles. To delimit the epileptic zone as precisely as possible, some recording electrodes (or at least some leads) needed to be localized outside the limits of the pathological zone. Consequently our present data were as much as possible gathered through recording from these presumably healthy or quasi-healthy brain sites. The identification of structures actually explored through the multiple recording sites was largely inferred from information provided by the SEEG staff, who systematically carried out electrical stimulation: single shocks were used to characterize the primary motor area, and repetitive shocks to identify the supplementary motor area [19, 20] and possibly also other areas (a conscious experience being reported by the patient when a given sensory area was stimulated).

All patients who accepted to participate in our recording sessions were amply informed that these sessions were not directly related to the search for their epileptic focus and had all given their consent. Our working sessions generally lasted between 60 and 90 min. For all recordings of the RPs and the CNVs (forewarned RT potential), the patients were comfortably lying in a bed and were instructed to fixate either a given point in the visual field or the videoscreen in front of them, depending on the test.

We used several types of CNV protocols. At the beginning, we used two acoustic stimuli, delivered through a loudspeaker: a first brief tone S1 (1,000 Hz, 75 dB, lasting 100 ms) as the warning stimulus, followed after 3 s (or sometimes only after 1.5 s) by the imperative stimulus S2 which was the repetition of similar tone bursts at 5/s. The subject was instructed to perform with one hand a movement (pressing a button) as rapidly as possible, to interrupt the S2 sequence. The successive trials with the S1–S2 sequence were delivered at random intervals around 10 s (10 ± 2 s). Blocks of 30 trials were recorded, with a fixed S1–S2 interval.

More recently, we changed our CNV paradigm in the following way: we kept the warning stimulus as a brief tone burst (this time at 400 Hz). The interval to the next imperative stimulus was still 1.5 s or more often 3 s, but S2 now consisted of visual patterns, briefly flashed for 100 ms on the videoscreen. The two patterns, a filled red circle or a red cross, had roughly the same luminance and were displayed in random order. With this second program, we adopted two distinct subprotocols. The first one was close to the classical CNV paradigm, in that the patient was instructed to perform a movement whenever the circle or the cross appeared (the requested movement was pressing on a joystick button) whereas in the second subprotocol, the instruction was to press the button only at appearance of the circle and to refrain from moving at that of the cross. This latter protocol is distinct from the classical go/no-go paradigm used in this type of studies, where the go or no-go instruction is given by the warning signal. Here also the intertrial interval was randomly fixed at 10 ± 2 s.

In the RP paradigm, the patient was instructed to perform the same button press as above, but at his own rhythm (at will, 'self-paced'). He was asked to maintain intervals of at least 10 s between successive movements, without counting or otherwise estimating the time. In cases of a unilateral motor deficit, the movements were all performed with the unaffected side.

All recordings from deep leads were performed against binaural reference electrodes. With this arrangement, the recording impedance was of a few thousand ohms. Surface electromyograms (EMGs) were recorded from a pair of cup electrodes placed on the skin over the flexor digitorum communis. Very often, we could record both the CNVs (30 tests with obligatory movements, 30 with go/no-go), and 30–50 RPs. Sometimes, for some reasons (lack of time, patient somewhat tired, etc.) we had to limit our study to the two CNV paradigms.

Data acquisition and averaging was obtained, using either a Nihon Kohden Neuropack 4 set with a bandpass from 0.01 to 500 Hz or, more recently a 32-channel EEG recorder fed into a CED 1401 interface with the 'SIGAV' software. In the CNV paradigm, averaging was started 500 ms before the S1 stimulus. In the RP paradigm, EMG onset was used for averaging (4 s pretrigger and 1 s posttrigger).

Results

We summarize several classes of results gained under various conditions. Rather than providing a systematic account, we shall consider here some salient observations concerning the slow potentials in relation to the motor performance of the patient.

General Features of the Recorded RPs and CNVs: Polarity and Shape

Whereas scalp-recorded CNVs were systematically negative when recorded monopolarly (fig. 1A), the morphology of the intracerebral CNV potentials varied considerably, between patients and between recording sites. In general the 'CNV-like' potentials (as we shall term them from now on) were suprisingly small, as compared to the scalp CNVs and also to the RPs which will be considered below. When they were present, they appeared bilaterally with similar amplitudes, not depending on the side of the moving limb. The large variability thus prevented any systematic classification. For example, in a patient we recorded (fig. 2A; CNV) a complex potential with a first positive shift, followed by a slowly increasing negative potential (measured slope: 50 μV/s), resembling a classical CNV, from the most mesial lead located in the supplementary motor area, SMA (M′1-1). More lateral

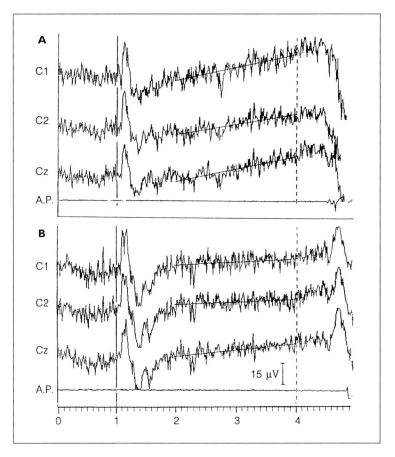

Fig. 1. CNV recorded from the scalp of a normal subject (P.B.). **A** Classical paradigm with a warning signal (tone, indicated by first cursor) followed after 3 s by an imperative stimulus (cross or circle pattern on videoscreen, indicated by second cursor). Notice evoked potential to the warning sound, followed by a slowly increasing CNV negativity (slope, ca. 15 μV/s) and then by an evoked potential roughly concomitant with the button pressing movement and developing thereafter as a large positive wave. **B** Paradigm with same warning stimulus, but the subject was asked to press the button only to one pattern (circle) and refrain from pressing to the other pattern (cross). Notice that 'CNV-like' potential is much smaller (slope at about 5 μV/s), the reaction time to the stimulus is longer (choice reaction time task) and the movement is preceded, at least in C2, by another slow potential with a steeper slope (about 15 μV/s) resembling a short-lasting RP. Upward deflection: negativity of the active electrode vs. mastoid reference (50 averaged records). C1 = Left central; C2 = right central; Cz = vertex; A.P. = EMG from active muscle.

leads (M'1-3), presumably recording from the white matter, detected the early positivity but not the late potentials. This early positivity may thus be part of the CNV, or rather, a late component of the evoked potential to the warning stimulus.

Another peculiar feature was the possible association of a CNV-like potential with an auditory evoked potential, when recording was performed from the vicinity of the

Heschl gyrus (fig. 2B). These potentials were of a classical type, comprising several components, the earliest probably being P100 (with the used time resolution, earlier components were hardly distinguishable). As we shall see below, more complex evoked potentials were recorded when we changed the protocol with the second stimulus now being a visual pattern.

Contrasting with the complexity of the potentials recorded in the warned reaction time task, the recorded RPs were of a more conventional shape and were generally fairly large (fig. 2A) and, except for their variable polarity, closer to the scalp-recorded ones (fig. 5). One of the problems raised by these potentials is whether the CNV-like potential, or at least its later part, is the equivalent of an RP. When comparing the two event-related potentials for their slopes, no conclusion could be drawn regarding the slope of the RP, compared to that of the end phase of the CNV-like potential.

Comparisons between RP and CNV Distributions

As emphasized earlier, both event-related potentials are very widely distributed over the scalp with only slight differences such as a larger amplitude of the RP on the contralateral side. The poor resolution of the scalp recording did not allow any precise localization. Contrastingly, intracerebral recordings provided more interesting data.

We could thus notice that the RP had a fairly limited distribution, being practically restricted to two brain sites, the premotor and motor cortex (MC) and the supplementary motor area (SMA). The MC was only activated in case of a contralateral movement while the SMA was so with contralateral as well as ipsilateral movement. No other point on the convexity was so far detected as a possible source for these potentials. More recently though, we were able to extend our observations somewhat and discover that RPs were also present in the two cingulate areas (fig. 3A).

The distribution of CNV-like potentials was somewhat broader than that of the RPs; they were mostly recorded from two cerebral regions, the central area, including again premotor and MC and postcentral parietal cortex, as well as the SMA and the underlying part of the cingulate gyrus (area 23 and 24). While RPs were only recorded contralaterally to the performed movement on the primary MC, CNVs were as a rule, bilateral (fig. 3B). Other areas were also active, such as the vicinity of the auditory area and, in 1 patient, the amygdala. In contrast, no slow potentials were recorded from structures like hippocampus and the hippocampal gyrus.

The S1–S2 Stimulation Paradigm: Comparison on the Classical Protocol versus
the 'Go/No-Go' One: The Post-S2 Visual Evoked Potentials (VEPs)

When using both protocols, several striking features were noticed: Firstly, we had expected that the resulting potentials would not be the same, depending on whether the subject was *preparing to move* to whichever S2 would appear (filled circle or cross pattern) or was *expecting* the second stimulus before deciding to either move or refrain from moving. In fact a clear difference between the classical paradigm and the go/no-go one was actually noticed in the scalp recordings of 1 of our control subjects (P.B.; compare fig. 1A to B). In our patients, the results were, however, very variable. As expected, their reaction times were as a rule longer in the go/no-go condition (choice reaction time task) than in the classical task, or when the patients were simply instructed to move at a visual signal, as shown in figure 4C1–C4 (simple reaction time task; compare fig. 4C3 with C4). All patients but 1 in our series of 15 developed a CNV-like potential (preceding S2) only when they knew that they had to move (classical CNV paradigm), and not in the go/no-go conditions

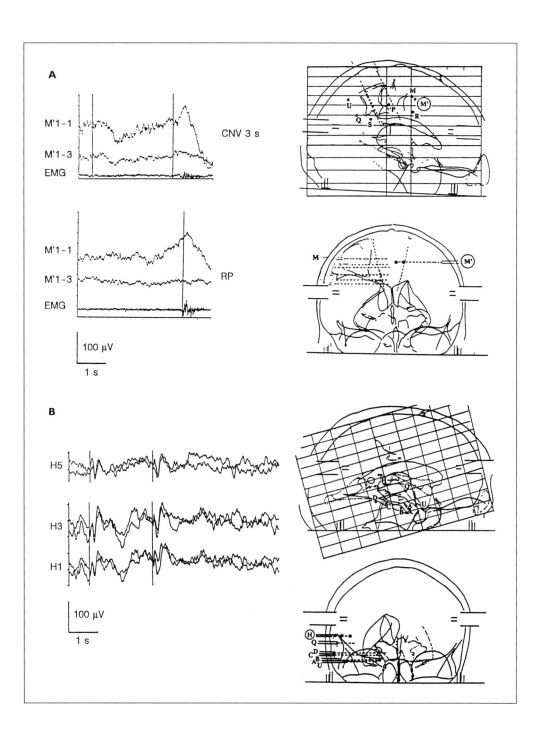

A

M'1−1

M'1−3

EMG

CNV 3 s

M'1−1

M'1−3

EMG

RP

100 µV

1 s

B

H5

H3

H1

100 µV

1 s

(compare fig. 4A1 with A2). Only 1 patient always displayed the same potential, whichever condition, perhaps due to a different strategy.

Secondly, the premotor potentials in the choice reaction time task with the 'go' signal were generally preceded by a slow deflection similar to the late part of an RP; this was not visible with 'no-go' stimuli (compare fig. 4B1 to B2). Thirdly, some differences were observed between the VEPs in case of movement (S2 obligatory or S2 go) and the no movement condition (S2 no-go), especially for some late components that tended to be larger when the subject performed a movement (see fig. 4C1–C4). This difference is likely due to the fact that motor potentials are added to the VEP itself, when a movement is performed. It was striking, however, that some VEP late components were even present in the no-go condition, as compared to the VEP obtained from the same subjects at the begining of the session, while they simply watched the visual stimulus (either cross or circle) before any pairing with sound or any instruction to move was given (compare fig. 4C1 with C2).

Special Features of the RPs

Interesting data were collected when examining some events preceding the RP, besides the classical progressive increase from the baseline starting at about 1,500 ms before the movement ('−1,500 ms').

(1) In 12 patients (out of 35), the execution of the movement was preceded by a transient event occurring at −2.2 to −3.0 s. These events resembled paroxystic interictal epileptic spikes. The striking feature was that the time interval between this event and the movement onset was almost constant in a given series of records. Hence, these events were visible on the averages. Actually it is on the averages that they were initially observed; since a contamination by high amplitude paroxysms or some artifact was suspected, the raw data were analyzed. In fact, due to their high amplitude in single records, overdrawing of these phasic events could be achieved (fig. 5). In other words, the RP may not be the first index of the preparation process of the movement, but may be preceded by phenomena that are normally covert and which may become visible under particular recording conditions. Scrutinizing the spontaneous ongoing activity in these patients showed that their tracing was somewhat perturbed, probably lying not very far from the ictal area. One may thus hypothesize that in this presumably hyperexcitable zone, such very discrete electrical

Fig. 2. A CNV-like and RP in patient with right centroparietal epileptic focus (30 averaged records). Same paradigm as figure 1A. Notice the difference in slope and duration between CNV and RP. Also note the amplitude difference between the lead close to the midline (M'1–1) and the more lateral one (M'1–3). M'1–1 = Left supplementary motor cortex; M'1–3 was 4.6 mm more lateral, presumably in the white matter. Each multilead electrode includes 1, 2 or 3 segments, each with 5 leads. The recording sites are designated by a letter and two numbers. For example, M'1–2 thus designates recording from second deepest lead on the first segment of left electrode M'. EMG = Muscle activity during right-hand movement. Localizations are indicated in sagittal (top) and frontal (bottom) X-ray views of the electrode placements [modified after 16]. **B** CNV-like potentials recorded from 3 leads at different levels in patients with right temporal epileptic focus within the right auditory cortex (H 5 being the most superficial). Two records, each corresponding to the movement of one hand are superimposed. Note strong similarity between traces for movements of left and right hand. The large positive deflection is only detected by the two deepest leads. In this specific case, the S1-S2 interval was 1.5 s. Same symbols as in **A** [from 16].

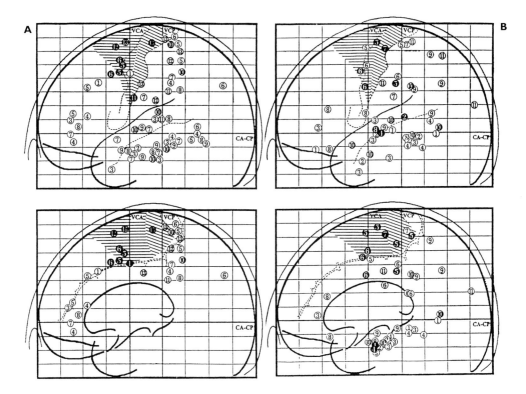

Fig. 3. A Overall topographical distribution of the recording electrodes in the explored cortex. Circles: points of entry of multilead depth electrodes, approaching from the lateral surface (top panel) and most often extending to the mesial surface (bottom panel). Numbers: numbers of patients. Filled circle: RP; empty circle: no RP. Horizontal hatching indicates precentral and premotor cortex and, on the mesial cortex, SMA; oblique hatching, hand and foot sensory areas. **B** Distribution of CNV-like potentials. Same display as in **A**. [From 16.]

events, revealing a very early process, may become overt while they are hardly or not visible in recordings from other more normal areas, and even more so, from the scalp. Another explanation, which is not antinomic to the preceding one, is that in these patients, movements precisely start to be prepared when a slight paroxystic event occurs within the time window of the programming of a volitional movement.

(2) Another rather spectacular feature was observed, that was somewhat similar to observations of Pfurtscheller and co-workers. Among our patients, many displayed high amplitude rhythms at about 8/s. Those could be considered as 'slow mu' rhythms, with their main functional characteristics of being interrupted about 2,000 ms before movement onset. This phenomenon was described by Pfurtscheller and Aranibar [21] under the term 'event-related desynchronization' (ERD). Our data tend to show that the initiation of the ERD with respect to movement onset occurs within the same temporal range as that of the RP in its conventional time evolution (fig. 6).

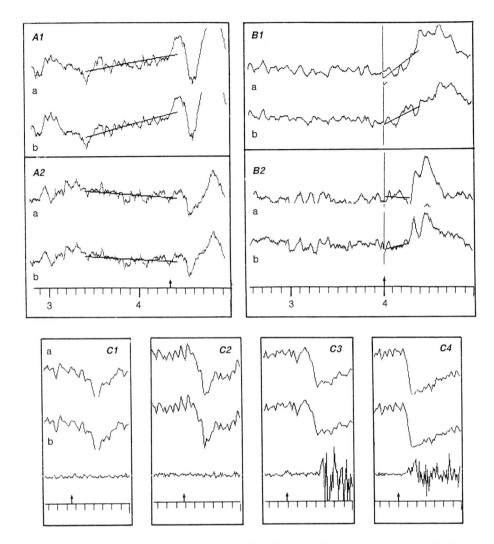

Fig. 4. Composite picture illustrating some salient features of the evoked potentials to the visual stimulus in a forewarned reaction time task with various protocols (see Methods). Records following the first, warning sound stimulus are not presented (20–30 averaged records). Time in s. Arrows: visual stimulus presentation. **A1–A2** A late CNV (negative) component is visible in the 'classical' CNV paradigm with the second, visual stimulus being imperative (**A1**) while no such event develops in the go/no-go paradigm (**A2**). a and b: records from two successive leads from one electrode situated in middle cingulate cortex. Patient (Ms Den.) with deep posterior temporal lesion. **B1–B2** ERPs recorded in two distinct conditions of the go/no-go paradigm: in **B1**, activity in go condition; in **B2**, activity in no-go condition. Notice absence of a classical CNV. On the other hand, an RP-like, short-lasting potential is visible when the patient, watching the go signal, takes a decision to move. In this patient (Ms Drou.) with a temporal epilepsy, records a and b were obtained from two leads, 4 mm apart, located in the depth of the central gyrus. **C1–C4** ERPs recorded in four distinct conditions. **C1**: visual stimulus applied without previous instruction (arrows); **C2** and **C3**: go/no-go conditions, with selected responses to no-go signal (**C2**) and to go signal (**C3**). **C4**: responses to visual stimulus, but used as instruction to move a joystick at stimulus (simple reaction time task). Patient (Mr Tar.) with temporal epilepsy. Two successive leads (a and b) were located in the depth of the posterior temporal lobe, in vicinity to the optic radiations. No CNV observed in this patient, but differences in amplitude of the late VEP component, when no movement was required from the patient. On bottom channel, EMG recording.

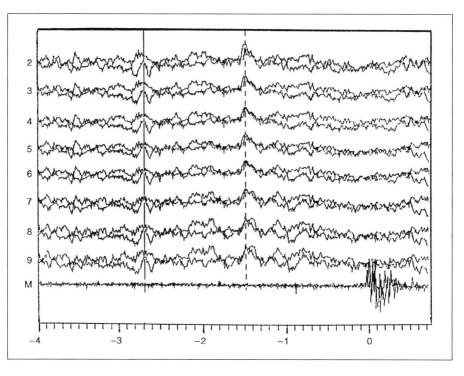

Fig. 5. Example of very early phasic events recorded in the RP paradigm. Instead of averaging, two successive trials were overdrawn. Notice two such events reproducible from one trial to the next, one at −2,700 ms, the other at −1,500 ms before the self-paced movement. No clear RP appeared in these conditions without averaging. Patient with temporal epileptic focus. Recording was taken from an electrode traversing the white matter all the way to the posterior cingulate gyrus (lead 9, the most superficial, to lead 2, the deepest one). M = Myographic recording of the movement.

Discussion

When Does Preparation for a Movement Begin?

The classical observations by Kornhuber and Deecke [5] have clearly indicated that events preceding movement onset exist in the brain, and are revealed by the development of the RP. The significance of this precession has raised an interesting debate, when Libet [8] suggested, from his observations on normal subjects, that the subject became only aware of his willingness to move in the last 500 ms before moving, meaning that the early part of the RP (i.e. about 1,000 ms) was an unconscious process. These conclusions have been amply discussed and sometimes challenged by others. We have no personal data to throw into this debate, but only the indication that the very first events in movement preparation (i.e. transient, 'phasic' events) may occur even earlier than the first part of the RP. We cannot however choose between the two not mutually exclusive explanations indicated above: (1) either that exploring a cortex which is particularly excitable, one may be able to detect an early phenomenon which remains covert to our recording procedure in more normal structures, even more so in scalp recordings, or (2) that the patient (as practically all subjects), despite the instruction not to count nor to be regular in determining

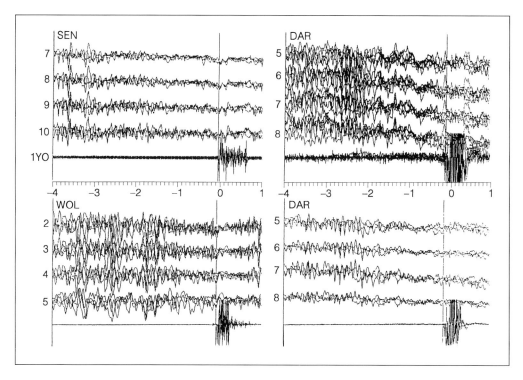

Fig. 6. Early desynchronization preceding self-paced movement with the right hand in 3 patients. All tracings were overdrawn to show constancy of these phenomena in successive recordings. In standard averages, such events did not appear clearly. Rhythms were in all 3 patients in the range of 7–8 Hz. Patients SEN and DAR: recordings from the deep parietal cortex; patient WOL, in the vicinity of SMA. Records taken from the left side. M and numbers: see legend to figure 5.

the movement onset, unavoidably adopts an approximate, rough timing of his movement (according to some kind of internal clock). In case of the patient with a cortex that is supernormally excitable, one may hypothesize that it is when, and perhaps only when a phasic event occurs during this time window, that the preparation of the movement begins.

Another indication that some events precede the movement itself was indeed given by Pfurtscheller and Aranibar [21] who described the ERD preceding for instance a finger movement. According to these authors, the ERD roughly displays the same time course as the classical RP described by Kornhuber and Deecke [5, their fig. 2]. All in all, our intracortical observations (fig. 6) roughly agree with these data, since they indicate that rhythm suppression precedes movement by 2 s, i.e. within the same time range as the RP. A result which is distinct from the above observation is the very early occurrence of phasic events in the movement programming in some other patients (fig. 5). These rhythms, as they were obtained in our patients, were slower than those usually described as 'mu rhythms', perhaps because these patients were under anticonvulsant therapy. On the other hand, it is very unlikely that they correspond to faster rhythms, first described by Jasper and Penfield [22], termed beta, and recently investigated by Pfurtscheller et al. [23].

About the Spatial Distribution of the Intracerebral CNVs and RPs

A striking feature is the contrast between the wide distribution of scalp RPs as well as CNVs, and the rather limited number of structures that displayed an intracerebral RP or CNV in our data. Clearly, the RPs mainly concern the contralateral primary motor area, the contralateral premotor area and the supplementary motor areas of both sides. The parietal cortex was only slightly active, while the temporal cortices remained silent (temporal convexity, deep limbic strutures such as amygdala, hippocampus and hippocampal gyrus). Nor did the prefrontal areas display any potential. In our 1994 publication [15] we also reported on the silence of the anterior cingulate cortex; since then we have been able to observe some RPs in this area (an observation that may be of interest given the potential functional importance recently lent to this structure by several groups). Some of the areas that are currently thought to be involved in the motor preparation or programming (e.g. the parietal or prefrontal cortex) were surprisingly silent when tested for the presence of an RP. One of the reasons of this absence may be the extreme simplicity and perfectly stereotyped character of the requested movement, which may not require any complex programming operation. This restricted localization of the cortical RPs also contradicts data in monkeys according to which RP-like potentials are present not only in the motor cortex, but also in the prefrontal and/or premotor and somatosensory cortices [24, 25].

We could also confirm observations, made with subdural and epidural recording, of RPs in the contralateral MC and bilateral SMAs [26, 27]. On the other hand, we failed to confirm the presence of an RP in the ipsilateral MC, as claimed by the latter groups.

The CNV-like potentials displayed some remarkable features: one is their limited extent, though somewhat larger than that of the RP, since some CNV-like potentials could also be recorded from the temporal lobe. The second is the small amplitude which generally characterized these potentials, as compared to the scalp ones. No such marked amplitude differences between scalp and intracerebral potentials were observed in case of the RPs. It may be that, in case of the CNV, the scalp plays an essential role as a spatial integrator.

A difficult point also emerged from these data: namely that we could not distinguish, in our records, the successive components in the RP and in the CNV, as were described by others. Based on scalp recordings, two distinct phases were separated in the standard CNV. The second part has been considered equivalent to an RP by several authors [see 11]. Our results with intracerebral recording do not allow comparison based on shapes of the potentials, given their variability. On the other hand, the anatomical distribution of CNV-like potentials tends to support the alternative opinion [12, 13] that the late part of the CNV cannot only be identified as an RP. One of the reasons might be that the spatial distribution of CNV potentials is somewhat larger than that of the RPs. All in all, we have so far been unable to answer the question whether the late component of the CNV shares the same generators as the RP. The observation that the distribution of the CNV-like potentials was somewhat broader than that of the Rps is only a partial answer. One of the explanations for this difference could be the presence, in the CNV late component (but not in the RP), of a potential described by some authors [see 14] as a 'stimulus preceding negativity' whose distribution would then mainly include the temporal areas.

Examining the Post-Second Stimulus Events in the Two Stimuli Protocols

One of our interests was concentrated on the shape of the event-related potentials to the second stimulus, when the latter was a visual pattern. That these components are not simply due to a reafference originating from the movement itself is indicated by their presence even in the no-go condition. Rather, they may belong to the family of 'intrinsic' components which, as has been well documented by many groups [see e.g. 28, 29], are significantly enhanced in situations requesting attentiveness: in fact these components were absent in our series when the visual stimulus was insignificant (fig. 4). One may thus conclude that these paradigms with a warning stimulus, even followed by a nonimperative stimulus, but involving perception and decision making, provide a particularly favorable condition to analyze attention processes. More data are, however, needed to reach conclusions on the spatiotemporal distribution of these potentials.

Acknowledgments

Some of the observations reported herein were carried out in collaboration with Dr. Ivan Rektor from the Clinic of Neurology, Masaryk University, Brno, Czech Republik. We wish to express our gratitude to Prof. Chodkiewicz and to the Ste Anne Hospital Neurosurgical staff. We also extend our thanks to Drs F. Chassoux and E. Landré for their valuable help, as well as to Dominique Chagot and Jean-Paul Gagnepain for assisting us during the recording sessions.

References

1   Walter WG, Cooper R, Aldridge VJ, McCallum C, Cohen J: The contingent negative variation: An electro-cortical sign of sensorimotor association in man. Electroencephalogr Clin Neurophysiol 1964;17:340–341.
2   Timsit-Berthier M: Variation contingente négative et composantes endogènes du potentiel évoqué. Rev EEG Neurophysiol Clin 1984;14:77–86.
3   Brunia CHM: Brain potentials related to preparation and action; in Heuer H, Sanders AF (eds): Perspectives in Preparation and Action. Hillsdale, Erlbaum, 1987, pp 105–130.
4   Böcker KBE, Forget R, Brunia CHM: The modulation of somatosensory evoked potentials during the fore-warned reaction time task. Electroencephalogr Clin Neurophysiol 1993;88:105–117.
5   Kornhuber HH, Deecke L: Hirnpotentialänderungen beim Menschen vor und nach Willkürbewegungen, darge-stellt mit Magnetbandspeicherung und Rückwärtsanalyse. Pflügers Arch 1964;281:52.
6   Kristeva R, Keller L, Deecke L, Kornhuber HH: Cerebral potentials preceding unilateral and simultaneous bilateral finger movements. Electroencephalogr Clin Neurophysiol 1979;47:229–238.
7   Shibasaki K, Barrett G, Halliday E, Halliday AM: Components of the movement-related cortical potential and their scalp topography. Electroencephalogr Clin Neurophysiol 1981;52:507–516.
8   Libet B: Unconscious cerebral initiative and the role of conscious will in voluntary action. Behav Brain Sci 1985;8:529–566.
9   Brunia CHM, Damen EJP: Distribution of slow brain potentials related to motor preparation and stimulus anticipation in a time estimation task. Electroencephalogr Clin Neurophysiol 1988;69:234–243.
10 Tarkka IM, Hallett M: Cortical topography of premotor and motor potentials preceding self-paced, voluntary movement of dominant and non-dominant hands. Electroencephalogr Clin Neurophysiol 1990;75:36–43.
11 Grünewald G, Grünewald-Zuberbier E, Netz J, Hömberg V, Sander G: Relationships between the late component of the contingent negative variation and the Bereitschaftspotential. Electroencephalogr Clin Neurophysiol 1979; 46:538–545.
12 Ruchkin DS, Sutton S, Mahaffey D, Glaser J: Terminal CNV in the absence of motor response. Electroencephalogr Clin Neurophysiol 1986;63:445–463.
13 Frost BG, Neill RA, Fenelon B: The determinants of the non-motoric CNV in a complex, variable foreperiod, information processing paradigm. Biol Psychol 1988;27:1–21.
14 Böcker KBE, Brunia CHM, van den Berg-Lennsen MM: A spatiotemporal dipole model of the stimulus preceding negativity prior to feedback stimuli. Brain Topogr 1994;7:71–88.
15 Rektor I, Fève A, Buser P, Bathien N, Lamarche M: Intracerebral recording of movement-related readiness potentials: An exploration in epileptic patients. Electroencephalogr Clin Neurophysiol 1994;90:273–283.
16 Lamarche M, Louvel J, Buser P, Rektor I: Intracerebral recordings of slow potentials in a contingent negative variation paradigm: An exploration in epileptic patients. Electroencephalogr Clin Neurophysiol 1995;95:268–276.
17 Talairach J, Szikla G, Tournoux P, Prossalentis A, Bordas-Ferrer M, Covello L: Atlas d'Anatomie Stéréotaxique du Télencéphale. Paris, Masson, 1967.
18 Talairach J, Tournoux P: Co-Planar Stereotaxic Atlas of the Human Brain. Stuttgart, Thieme, 1988.
19 Penfield W, Welch K: The supplementary motor area of the cerebral cortex. Arch Neurol Psychiatry 1951;66: 289–317.

20 Talairach J, Bancaud J: The supplementary motor area in man. J Neurol 1966;5:330–347.
21 Pfurtscheller G, Aranibar A: Evaluation of event-related desynchronization preceding and following voluntary self-paced movements. Electroencephalogr Clin Neurophysiol 1979;46:138–146.
22 Jasper H, Penfield W: Electrocorticograms in man: Effect of the voluntary movement upon the electrical activity of the precentral gyrus. Arch Psychiatr Z Neurol 1949;183:163–173.
23 Pfurtscheller G, Pregenzer M, Neuper C: Visualization of sensorimotor areas involved in preparation for hand movement based on classification of mu and beta rhythms in single EEG trials in man. Neurosci Lett 1994; 181:43–46.
24 Gemba H, Hashimoto S, Sasaki K: Slow potentials preceding self-paced hand movements in the parietal cortex of monkeys. Neurosci Lett 1979;15:87–92.
25 Sasaki K, Gemba H, Hashimoto S: Premovement slow potentials on self-paced movements and thalamocortical and corticocortical responses in the monkey. Exp Neurol 1981;72:41–50.
26 Neshige R, Lueders H, Shibasaki H: Recording of movement-related potentials from scalp and cortex in man. Brain 1988, 111:719–736.
27 Ikeda A, Lueders H, Burgess R, Shibasaki H: Movement-related potentials recorded from supplementary motor area and primary motor area: Role of supplementary motor area in voluntary movements. Brain 1992;115: 1017–1043.
28 Hillyard S, Kutas M: Electrophysiology of cognitive processes. Annu Rev Psychol 1983;34:33–61.
29 Hillyard S: Electrophysiology of human selective attention. Trends Neurosci 1986;8:400–405.

Dr. Pierre Buser, Institut des Neurosciences, Université P. et M. Curie,
9, Quai St. Bernard, F–75005 Paris Cedex 05 (France)

Hepp-Reymond M-C, Marini G (eds): Perspectives of Motor Behavior and Its Neural Basis.
Basel, Karger, 1997, pp 91–102

....

Transcranial Brain Stimulation for Studying the Human Motor System

C. W. Hess, J. Mathis, K. M. Rösler, R. Müri

University Department of Neurology, Inselspital, Bern, Switzerland

Since the pioneering work of Fritsch and Hitzig [1], who examined the exposed motor cortex of dogs with direct electrical stimuli producing limb movements, brain stimulation has been a classical instrument to investigate the mammalian motor system in experimental neurophysiology. The neocortical motor areas of monkeys were subsequently explored in detail by electrical stimulation of the cortex by Ferrier [2] and Horsley [3]. Also in the last century, direct faradic cortical stimulation of the exposed human motor cortex was applied by surgeons during cranial operations, and this has later become a standard method for localizing the precentral gyrus during neurosurgery. However, only with the introduction of transcranial cortical stimulation in the 1980s by Merton and Morton [4], has the clinical neurophysiologist been given a tool to assess the human motor system in the intact subject. Merton used single high-voltage electric shocks from a large capacitor to penetrate the scalp and skull and successfully excited the motor or visual cortex causing contralateral muscle twitches or phosphenes, respectively. Like Fritsch and Hitzig [1], Merton and Morton [4] achieved motor responses most easily with the anode over the motor area, and this has been explained by the formation of virtual cathodes within or beneath the grey matter where it excites the pyramidal neurones at the axon hillock.

A major drawback of the transcranial electric stimulation in alert human subjects was the considerable local discomfort on the scalp, which limited its use in clinical and experimental work. This obstacle was ingeniously overcome by Pat Merton only 5 years later who used a stimulator devised by Barker et al. [5] which generated brief intense magnetic pulses. The single magnetic pulse induces stimulating currents directly within the brain causing only trivial scalp sensation.

Since single magnetic pulses over the scalp produce respectable limb jerks and sizeable muscle responses as recorded by surface EMG electrodes, no averaging is required and the simple recording procedure resembles very much that of peripheral neurography. The method has, therefore, gained broad acceptance among clinical neurophysiologists who eagerly awaited an easily applicable method to directly assess the pyramidal system. Transcranial magnetic stimulation (TMS) of the motor cortex has meanwhile proved to be of great value in the diagnosis of neurological disorders involving the pyramidal motor system. Marked latency prolongation is suggestive of demyelination of central motor pathways [6], whereas low-amplitude responses with little delay are more typical of disorders causing central axonal neuronal loss due to degeneration [7]. Subclinical abnormalities in

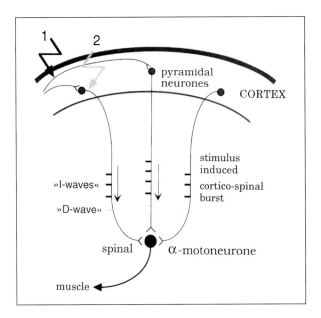

Fig. 1. Schematic graph on the presumed dominant stimulation site and mechanism of excitation of the spinal motoneurones by transcranial magnetic (1) and transcranial anodal electrical (2) motor cortex stimulation.

the pyramidal motor system may be demonstrated [8], and the technique has a potential role for quantification of disease progress.

Basic Features of the Motor-Evoked Responses

The most obvious effect of single pulse magnetic brain stimulation is a motor-evoked response (MER) which, by nature of its short latency, must be conveyed by the rapidly conducting pyramidal system and by monosynaptic excitatory connections with the motoneurones [9]. However, additional activation of both slowly conducting or indirect as well as inhibitory motor pathways cannot be precluded and have in fact been partly disclosed [10, 11]. As was shown in early animal work [12], and has also been demonstrated in humans, a single cortical shock sets up a short train of descending impulses in the pyramidal fibers [13, 14] allowing for spatial and temporal summation of excitatory postsynaptic potentials in the bulbar and spinal motoneurones which are known to require several excitatory postsynaptic potentials to reach firing threshold (fig. 1). A conspicuous feature of the MERs is its facilitation by a voluntary effort directed towards the target muscle. Slight voluntary contraction produces responses with greater amplitudes and shorter latencies. The mechanism of this facilitation probably resides on spinal as well as cortical level (see below).

Interestingly, a marked latency difference between the MERs of the TMS technique and the anodal electrical stimulation was found, the latter producing responses with 2–3 ms shorter onset latencies [9]. This raises the question as to the excited neural structures responsible for the MERs when using the two stimulating techniques (fig. 1). Although the question still awaits ultimate clarification, one has good reasons to assume that, with moderate stimulus intensities, the magnetic stimulus predominantly excites neural elements in the cortex which are presynaptic to the pyramidal cells, whereas the anodal electric stimulus additionally excites the pyramidal cells directly, thus inducing shorter onset latencies [15]. However, regardless of the stimulus modality used, one should always bear in mind that with transcranial stimulation, neural elements other than the target circuitry are also activated. Given the highly refined and extremely complex structure and function of the human brain, the coarse transcranial magnetoelectric stimulus contrasts with the delicate techniques of experimental motor cortex microstimulation in animals. Although efforts to develop stimulating coils with a more focal stimulus proved successful [16], the cortical region subjected to the stimulus is bound to be relatively extended, and this obviously limits the technique in experimental work. Since the stimulus cannot be confined to a specific target structure in the brain, a great variety of different neural elements are inevitably excited, some of which have excitatory and others probably inhibitory action. On the other hand, TMS has the great advantage of being applicable in the conscious and cooperating subject thus allowing interfering paradigms during sophisticated motor tasks.

Facilitation of Motor Responses by Voluntary and Involuntary Preinnervation

The threshold for evoking motor responses is markedly reduced, the amplitude enhanced, and the onset latency shortened when the TMS is applied during a voluntary contraction of the target muscle [9]. The precise mechanisms of this facilitation by preactivation is not yet known in detail and might be different depending on the target muscle under study. However, a spinal mechanism seems likely. Amplitudes of MERs enlarge with increasing voluntary background contraction (fig. 2), and the exact relation between amplitude and background contraction depends on the stimulus strength and differs from muscle to muscle [17]. Conversely, the latency shortening of the MER when changing from relaxed to active state of the target muscle does not change any further with increasing background contraction nor does it differ much between various muscles [16]. It could be explained by an increased synaptic efficacy on spinal level: during subliminal activation less temporal summation of impinging excitatory impulses of the descending volley is needed and the motoneurones reach firing threshold earlier. The facilitation-induced latency shortening of individual motor units as recorded by needle electrodes is in fact not a continuous one but is jumping in discrete steps of approximately 1.2–1.5 ms which matches the interspike intervals of the descending pyramidal volleys [18]. Consequently, the facilitation-induced latency shortening has been shown to be absent when the spinal cord is stimulated directly, since this induces only one descending impulse in the corticospinal fibers [19].

Since voluntary activation of the target muscle facilitates the MER, it was interesting to see whether involuntary muscle activation would also have a similar facilitating effect on MERs and to what degree. If we relate the amplitudes of stimulus-induced responses of the deltoid muscle to the degree of voluntary background contraction, we get a linear dependence, and this is also true for reflexively induced background contraction, e.g. by vibration of the tendon. We also used the 'postcontraction phenomenon' of Konstamm (fig. 3A), where the subject has to exert a strong volitional abducting effort with his arm against resistance for several minutes prior to the cortical stimulus. When subsequently

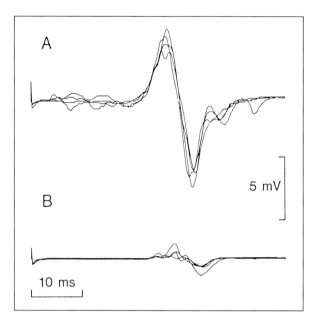

Fig. 2. Effect of voluntary background contraction on stimulus-induced responses as recorded from the hypothenar muscle of the hand: Compound muscle action potentials (**A**) during voluntary background contraction and (**B**) from a completely relaxed muscle. The responses were obtained with identical stimulus intensity and coil position on the scalp (several responses superimposed). Note the greater amplitude and shorter onset latency during preinnervation (**A**), and the inherent variability in both conditions.

relaxing, the arm will perform an involuntary abduction which is believed to be of subcortical origin. The cortical stimulus is given during the involuntary contraction (fig. 3B), and we find the same linear relation as with voluntary contraction, thus corroborating the idea of spinal origin of this facilitation. We thus assume that for proximal muscles most of the facilitation occurs on spinal level.

Investigating the Rapid Corticospinal Tract in Humans

The MERs also allow us to study in man simple but clinically important questions about the functional motor organization, which experiments in animals cannot resolve because of significant differences among species. The sequelae of pyramidal tract lesions in patients and subsequent repair of function are clinically relevant questions which are not yet fully understood [20]. Furthermore, it was not known whether proximal limb muscles and trunk muscles are being controlled also by the rapidly conducting corticospinal routes. And the question whether a skeletal muscle's motoneurone pool is innervated unilaterally or bilaterally by the rapidly conducting monosynaptic corticobulbar and corticospinal routes has great impact on clinical work. Until now, only indirect evidence from stroke or tumor lesions was available, and for many proximal and axial muscle no clear-cut picture emerged regarding its rapid pyramidal supply.

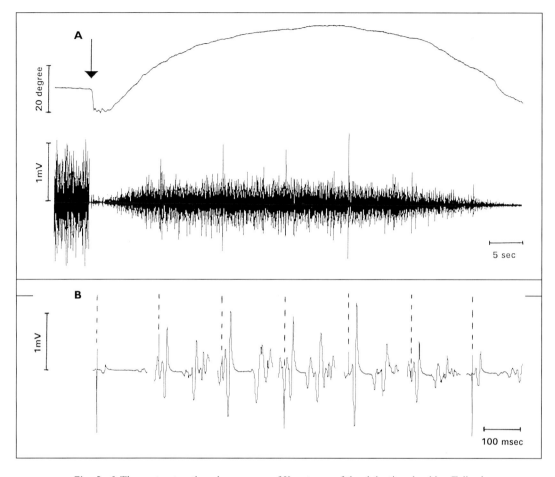

Fig. 3. A The postcontraction phenomenon of Konstamm of the abducting shoulder: Following a forceful abduction against resistance, the deltoid muscle is relaxed (arrow), and an involuntary abduction lasting several seconds is exerted. Angle of shoulder abduction (upper trace) and surface recorded EMG activity of the deltoid muscle (lower trace) is shown. **B** Stimulus-induced MERs during the involuntary Konstamm contraction of figure 3A: Repeated recordings from the deltoid muscle while cortical stimuli are given (interrupted vertical lines). Note the increasing and waning amplitudes of MERs.

An important methodological prerequisite for this kind of study was the use of focal enough magnetic stimuli which are absolutely confined to one hemisphere. And with this respect some earlier studies using large circular stimulating coils with their great stimulus spread produced disputable results about purported unilateral corticospinal connections. Even by using the unpleasant anodal-electric technique, the stimulus spread cannot be safely prevented. With the development of figure-of-eight-shaped twin coils [16] this methodological limitation has been overcome also for magnetic stimulation, and we are now quite confident that with moderate stimulus intensities and appropriate coil position on the scalp a stimulus spread to the other hemisphere can safely be prevented.

The corticospinal projection to *proximal limb muscles* in man was repeatedly studied using cortical stimulation and poststimulus time histograms of motor units as recorded by needle electrodes [21, 22]. As expected, a very strong rapidly conducting monosynaptic corticospinal projection was found for the intrinsic hand muscles. Quite substantial, albeit weaker rapid monosynaptic projection was also disclosed for the forearm and biceps brachii muscles, and the shoulder muscles receive still weaker rapid corticospinal monosynaptic input [22]. Some short latency excitation in motor units of the deltoid and pectoralis major muscles was nevertheless demonstrated [21]. This confirms experiences from surface recordings of the deltoid muscle and using greater stimulus intensities which also produce short latency responses. Rather surprisingly, the external sphincter muscle was also found to be supplied by rapidly conducting corticospinal routes [23]. As with limb muscles, the MER of the external anal sphincter and bulbocavernosus muscles were facilitated by voluntary activation with a shortening of the onset latencies by about 5 ms. However, when comparing the MER of the sphincter with those of a lower limb muscle such as the tibialis anterior, the latency to the sphincter is longer by several milliseconds and, other than with limb muscles, the centrally evoked late responses (with a corticomuscular latency of around 100 ms) had a lower threshold than the short latency MER [23]. This was interpreted as indicating a polysynaptic transmission to the sphincter muscle. Motor cortex stimulation experiments have, furthermore, shown that the diaphragm can be activated by rapidly conducting oligosynaptic pathways [24]. With an average calculated central conduction time of 4.3 ms to the spinal motoneurones of the diaphragm, the corticospinal delay was similar to that for the deltoid muscle. Again, voluntary activation by inspiration facilitated the responses. Obviously, it is possible to bypass the brainstem respiratory centers by this rapid corticospinal route. While this was expected to be the case for the intercostal respiratory muscles, known to be much involved in speech production, this was not generally expected for the diaphragm which primarily serves respiration.

The situation proved more complex for the cranial muscles, where there is a considerable variance of onset latencies between the muscles suggesting distinct peculiarities of corticobulbar connections. The corticomuscular latency of the MERs from the facial muscles is approximately 10 ms [25], which is almost as much as the latency to the biceps brachii muscle (approx. 11 ms), the central and peripheral motor routes of which being much longer. Also, the MERs of the facial muscles require more facilitation by voluntary background contraction in order to be recordable. It is, therefore, a reasonable assumption that even the most rapidly conducting corticobulbar routes to the facial muscles are polysynaptic. On the other hand, with an onset latency to the masticatory muscles of only about 5.5 ms [26], a rapidly conducting oligo- or monosynaptic connection must be assumed for the latter muscles. These differences probably reflect the greater complexity of the central network serving the facial muscles as compared to that serving the masticatory muscles. The facial system with its refined and complicated mimic functions is bound to be more complex than the masticatory one.

For the facial muscles it also proved easy to demonstrate the existence of an important (uncrossed) ipsilateral corticobulbar supply, as might be expected from standard textbooks. However, quite unexpectedly, substantial ipsilateral corticobulbar supply was not only revealed for the most rostral part of facial muscles (e.g. m. frontalis) but in many subjects also for the lower facial muscles (fig. 4). This finding clearly contradicts the widely accepted neuroanatomical conception of exclusively crossed innervation of the lower facial muscles, producing the typical 'central facial pattern' following a unilateral central lesion with a paretic lower face and spared frontal muscles. The finding nevertheless meets the occasional

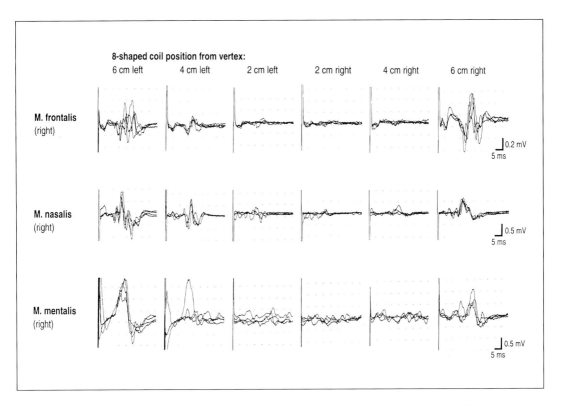

Fig. 4. MER from three right-sided facial muscles when moving the focal magnetic stimulus over the scalp from the left to the right facial motor cortex area. Several responses of the same coil position are superimposed. Ipsilateral (uncrossed) responses are recorded from the frontal muscle of similar amplitude than contralaterally, and also from the nasal and mental muscles albeit of somewhat smaller amplitudes than contralaterally. No responses can be recorded with the coil near the vertex invalidating the assumption of reflexive (e.g. trigeminofacial) responses.

clinical observation of a 'peripheral-type' facial palsy (comprising all parts of the facial muscles on one side) following a capsular stroke. Obviously there is a considerable, previously underestimated intersubject variation with this respect. Furthermore, we now have reason to assume that electrophysiologically revealed ipsilateral (uncrossed) corticospinal fibers must not necessarily become effective to the extent of being functionally apparent under a volitional effort when the dominant corticospinal supply from the contralateral side is interrupted. Also, in other cranial muscles such as masticatory [27, 28], lingual muscles [29], and accessory nerve innervated muscles [30], a variable short latency ipsilateral contribution was found. The situation is not that clear for proximal limb muscles where in some normal subjects ipsilateral MER could be demonstrated, the onset latencies of which being longer by several milliseconds than the latencies of the contralateral responses. Therefore, for these muscles, apart from uncrossed corticospinal routes, transcallosal transmission could be an alternative explanation for the ipsilateral MERs [31].

Plasticity of the Human Brain

Plasticity of the human brain is an issue of paramount clinical importance which can be investigated by magnetic brain stimulation. It has, for instance, been found that after a limb amputation, the excitable cortical representation of the remaining proximal muscles is expanding [32, 33], and this has been interpreted on the bases of structural reorganization of the central nervous system. Subsequent experiments on healthy subjects in Mark Hallet's laboratory [34] demonstrated rapidly reversible functional changes of human motor output to the biceps and thenar muscles after transient deafferentation of the forearm using a pneumatic cuff and regional anesthesia just below the elbow. Hence, functional plasticity may also play an important role under pathological conditions, and unmasking of inactive corticospinal connections was assumed in the case rapid functional changes. However, one should be careful in jumping to conclusions, and, at the present stage, we can only conclude that some corticospinal connections which cannot be evidenced by cortical stimulation under physiological conditions may be activated by stimulation under the artificial conditions of deafferentation. Furthermore, rapidly conducting uncrossed connections have been unveiled by MER in a variety of central neurological disorders. Animal studies from Mario Wiesendanger's laboratory [35] suggest that in monkeys ipsilateral corticospinal fibers could possibly participate in the functional recovery following pyramidal lesions. Several studies in patients following acute stroke demonstrating novel ipsilateral projections remain controversial for methodological reasons (see above). However, short latency ipsilateral pathways could be demonstrated beyond doubt in congenital mirror movements and in patients with hemispherectomy performed at an early age for intractable seizures [36].

Functional Inhibition

Magnetic brain stimulation also offers the possibility to produce *inhibitory effects*. An interesting example is the use of *transcallosal inhibition*. We know that the corpus callosum, among other functions, mediates important mutual inhibitory actions between analogous areas of the two hemispheres. However, the hand representation of the primary motor cortex is known to have poor callosal interconnection in mammals, and this has been shown to be true also in monkeys [37]. Therefore, the investigation of transcallosal connections of the hand area in humans, where dexterity is much more developed than in nonhuman primates and thus important differences might be expected, would be an area of great interest.

Using an appropriately timed cortical stimulus on one hemisphere virtually abolishes the MER in a hand muscle to a subsequent stimulus on the other side (fig. 5). Based on the timely relationship between the two stimuli and the presumed callosal conduction properties, we assume that the MER suppression is due to a stimulus-induced transcallosal inhibition. To test this hypothesis we used the technique in patients with a defective corpus callosum as shown by brain imaging studies. And the inhibitory effect was indeed lacking or reduced (fig. 5) in most of these patients thus corroborating the assumption of a transcallosal transmission. The method could thus be used to assess functional integrity of part of the corpus callosum in humans.

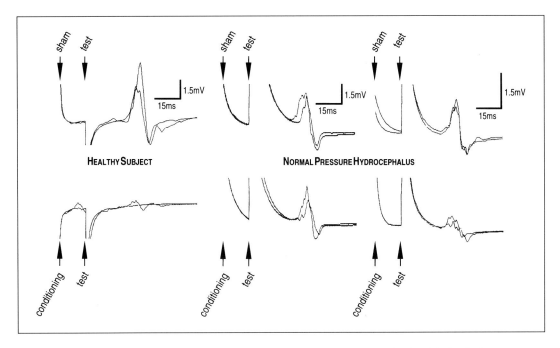

Fig. 5. Transcallosal inhibition using a conditioning cortical stimulus over the right hemisphere 14 ms prior to a test stimulus over the left hemisphere while recording from the hypothenar muscle of the right hand. In healthy subjects (left traces) the stimulus-induced MER is largely suppressed (lower trace left), whereas with empty trials using an inappropriately tuned sham conditioning shock and genuine test stimulus (upper trace) no suppression is observed. In a patient with a normal pressure hydrocephalus and severed corpus callosum the suppression of the MER is virtually lacking (middle and right lower traces), thus indicating insufficient callosal transmission of inhibitory impulses.

Cortical Stimulation for Interfering Paradigms in Humans

TMS enables the clinical neurophysiologist to excite the human brain in a fully alert and cooperating subject allowing to interfere with simple and complex conscious action. Both stimulus placement on the scalp as well as stimulus intensities must be very carefully tuned in order to optimally hit a target area without unnecessary stimulus spread. Because of the complexity of the implied central processing and uncertainties about the stimulated neural elements, the explanation of stimulating effects remains difficult. Brain stimulation to interfere with motor tasks is perhaps the most pretentious application of TMS, and the interpretation of its effects should be very cautious. Because of its precise timing, the method can nevertheless give valuable information which is complementary to functional imaging techniques with their limited time resolution. Although it has become possible to detect brain areas involved in motor tasks with functional imaging, the accurate timely sequence of the processing events in separate areas remains uncertain. Electrical or magnetic brain mapping with their unequalled time resolution often do not produce unequivocal results in terms of identifying 'active' brain areas. If one is successful in evidencing an exclusive vulnerable time window during which a motor task can be disturbed by TMS, and this is only possible when applying a focal stimulus at a certain site over the brain without effect when stimulating elsewhere, one may be fairly confident to deal with a specific result related to the task studied. Interference by a brain stimulus may delay the execution of a motor task or render its performance inaccurate, and direct or indirect activation of inhibitory neural elements of the target circuitry may then be assumed. If, on the contrary, the execution is precipitated by the stimulus, activation excitatory neural elements of the target circuitry would seem likely.

Rothwell et al. [38] used appropriately timed brain stimuli during voluntary movement of the wrist in response to an auditory signal and thus produced a delay of the movement of up to 150 ms, without affecting the motor pattern as such. We investigated the oculomotor system using various interfering paradigms, since we did not obtain direct oculomotor responses by TMS. It also proved very difficult to disturb the saccadic system by single cortical shocks when using direct visually guided saccades. Such direct saccades are assumed to use the midbrain rather than cortical oculomotor centers. Using an antisaccadic paradigm in order to avoid visual reflex elicitation, it proved possible to prolong saccadic latency by frontal TMS when the stimuli were applied during a narrow vulnerable time period which varied from subject to subject. In this paradigm, the subject was presented with laterally positioned targets which light up on one side, but he was instructed to look to the opposite side as quickly as possible [39]. Such a performance is very likely involving cortical processing, and the frontal eye field might well be the crucial structure. We subsequently applied TMS over the presumed supplementary motor eye field during performance of memorized sequences of saccades. The number of errors in executing the saccades increased significantly if the TMS was given 80 ms before or 60 ms after the 'go' signal [40]. There was no increase in errors when the coil was positioned over the occipital cortex, or when the stimulator output was too low (empty trials). With this paradigm, TMS probably interfered with the function of the supplementary eye field during a vulnerable time interval after the 'go' signal. Furthermore, following experiments comparing left and right parietal stimulation suggests a hemispheric functional asymmetry in the control of eye movements: other than the right posterior parietal cortex, the left was one not vulnerable during the same paradigm of memorized saccades [41]. This lateralization of the cortical control of saccades indicating a dominant right posterior parietal region comes as a surprise. It offers an analogy of the cortically guided eye movements with the dexterity of skilled hand movements with their well-known left-sided cortical dominance. Obviously, highly advanced and complex cortical functions of the human brain are best achieved by specializing into one hemisphere.

Conclusions

TMS of the human cortex is a simple and well-tolerated procedure which is now widely used by clinical neurophysiologists to assess the integrity of the central motor pathways in neurological disorders. Apart from its clinical use, the method has proved to be a particularly valuable tool to investigate the physiology of the human motor system. It has allowed some important insight into the functional organization of the 'pyramidal' motor system, where it enabled us to elucidate specific patterns of corticospinal and corticobulbar projections. Several magnetic stimulation studies in normal subjects and in patients investigated the plasticity of the human brain and make it look a very promising tool for further research in this field. Finally, since TMS is lacking any discomfort and can be used in the cooperating subject, it was possible, by using interfering paradigms, to unveil the timely sequence of brain processing during some complex motor tasks. In this respect, magnetic brain stimulation is complementary to the functional imaging techniques, with their higher spatial but poor temporal resolution. We have great hope that in the future magnetic stimulation in combination with imaging will help us to give important cues for a better understanding of the compensating mechanisms in an injured or diseased human brain. It is even conceivable that neurological rehabilitation strategies will at some time be individually tailored according to findings collected from magnetic stimulation studies.

One major limitation of the method lies in the limited focality of the stimulus within the brain in spite of important methodical improvements in this respect. However, there is still a considerable potential for further development of this relatively novel method. Only recently has it also become possible to apply double and even multiple transcranial magnetic stimuli. Rapid rate magnetic stimulation over the brain enhances considerably its efficacy, and it has already been used for experimental studies in human subjects [42]. The greater efficacy is, however, achieved at the expense of some important values and advantages: it abates its temporal punctuality, makes it a bit uncomfortable, and is not quite free of side effects. But there is ample room for technical improvement, and much of the mentioned drawbacks will hopefully be overcome in due course.

References

1   Fritsch G, Hitzig E: Ueber die elektrische Erregbarkeit des Grosshirns. Arch Anat Physiol Wiss Med (Leipzig) 1870;37:300–332.
2   Ferrier D: Experiments on the brain of monkeys. Proc R Soc Lond 1875;23:409–430.
3   Horsley V: A note on the means of topographical diagnosis of focal disease affecting the so-called motor region of the cerebral cortex. Am J Med Sci 1887;93:342–369.
4   Merton PA, Morton HB: Stimulation of the cerebral cortex in the intact human subject. Nature 1980;285: 227.
5   Barker AT, Freeston JL, Jalinous R, Merton PA, Morton HB: Magnetic stimulation of the human brain. J Physiol (Lond) 1985;369:3P.
6   Hess CW, Mills KR, Murray NMF: Measurement of central motor conduction in multiple sclerosis by magnetic brain stimulation. Lancet 1986;ii:355–358.
7   Schriefer TN, Hess CW, Mills KR, Murray NM: Central motor conduction studies in motor neurone disease using magnetic brain stimulation. Electroencephalogr Clin Neurophysiol 1989;74:431–437.
8   Hess CW, Mills KR, Murray NMF, Schriefer TN: Magnetic brain stimulation: Central motor conduction studies in multiple sclerosis. Ann Neurol 1987;22:744–752.
9   Hess CW, Mills KR, Murray NMF: Responses in small hand muscles from magnetic stimulation of the human brain. J Physiol (Lond) 1987;388:397–412.
10 Fuhr P, Agostino R, Hallett M: Spinal motor neuron excitability during the silent period after cortical stimulation. Electroencephalogr Clin Neurophysiol 1991;81:257–262.
11 Mills KR: Excitatory and inhibitory effects on human spinal motoneurones from magnetic brain stimulation. Neurosci Lett 1988;94:297–302.
12 Kernell D, Wu CP: Responses of the pyramidal tract to stimulation of the baboon's motor cortex. J Physiol (Lond) 1967;191:653–672.
13 Berardelli A, Inghilleri M, Cruccu G, Manfredi M: Descending volley after electrical and magnetic transcranial stimulation in man. Neurosci Lett 1990;112:54–58.
14 Thompson PD, Day BL, Crockard HA, Calder I, Murray NM, Rothwell JC, Marsden CD: Intra-operative recording of motor tract potentials at the cervico-medullary junction following scalp electrical and magnetic stimulation of the motor cortex. J Neurol Neurosurg Psychiatry 1991;54:618–623.
15 Day BL, Dressler D, Maertens de Noordhout A, Marsden CD, Nakashima K, Rothwell JC, Thompson PD: Electric and magnetic stimulation of human motor cortex: Surface EMG and single motor unit responses. J Physiol (Lond) 1989;412:449–473.
16 Rösler KM, Hess CW, Heckmann R, Ludin HP: Significance of shape and size of the stimulating coil in magnetic stimulation of the human motor cortex. Neurosci Lett 1989;100:347–352.
17 Kischka U, Fajfr R, Fellenberg T, Hess CW: Facilitation of motor evoked potentials from magnetic brain stimulation in man: A comparative study of different target muscles. J Clin Neurophysiol 1993;10: 505–512.

18 Hess CW, Mills KR, Murray NMF: Entladungscharakteristika der durch transkranielle Kortexreizung aktivi-erten motorischen Einheiten in den Handmuskeln des Menschen. Z EEG-EMG 1988;19:216–221.

19 Maertens de Noordhout A, Pepin JL, Gerard P, Delwaide PJ: Facilitation of responses to motor cortex stimulation: Effects of isometric voluntary contraction. Ann Neurol 1992;32:365–370.

20 Wiesendanger M: Pyramidal tract function and the clinical 'pyramidal syndrome'. Hum Neurobiol 1984;2: 227–234.

21 Colebatch JG, Day BL, Marsden CD, Rothwell JC, Thompson PD: Cortical outflow to proximal arm muscles in man. Brain 1990;113:1843–1856.

22 Palmer E, Ashby P: Corticospinal projections to upper limb motoneurones in humans. J Physiol (Lond) 1992; 448:397–412.

23 Ertekin C, Hansen MV, Larsson LE, Sjödahl R: Examination of the descending pathway to the external anal sphincter and pelvic floor muscles by transcranial cortical stimulation. Electroencephalogr Clin Neurophysiol 1990;75:500–510.

24 Gandevia SC, Rothwell JC: Activation of the human diaphragm from the motor cortex. J Physiol (Lond) 1987; 384:109–118.

25 Rösler KM, Hess CW, Schmid UD: Investigation of facial motor pathways by electrical and magnetic stimulation: Sites and mechanisms of excitation. J Neurol Neurosurg Psychiatry 1989;52:1149–1156.

26 Türk U, Rösler KM, Mathis J, Müllbacher W, Hess CW: Assessment of motor pathways to masticatory muscles: An examination technique using electrical and magnetic stimulation. Muscle Nerve 1994;17:1271–1277.

27 Cruccu G, Berardelli A, Inghilleri M, Manfredi M: Functional organization of the trigeminal motor system in man. A neurophysiological study. Brain 1989;112:1333–1350.

28 Carr LJ, Harrison LM, Stephens JA: Evidence for bilateral innervation of certain homologous motoneurone pools in man. J Physiol (Lond) 1994;475:217–227.

29 Muellbacher W, Mathis J, Hess CW: Electrophysiological assessment of central and peripheral motor routes to the lingual muscles. J Neurol Neurosurg Psychiatry 1994;57:309–315.

30 Berardelli A, Priori A, Inghilleri M, Cruccu G, Mercuri B, Manfredi M: Corticobulbar and corticospinal projections to neck muscle motoneurons in man. A functional study with magnetic and electric transcranial brain stimulation. Exp Brain Res 1991;87:402–406.

31 Wassermann EM, Fuhr P, Cohen LG, Hallett M: Effects of transcranial magnetic stimulation on ipsilateral muscles. Neurology 1991;41:1795–1799.

32 Cohen LG, Bandinelli S, Findley TW, Hallett M: Motor reorganization after upper limb amputation in man. A study with focal magnetic stimulation. Brain 1991;114:615–627.

33 Hall EJ, Flament D, Fraser C, Lemon RN: Non-invasive brain stimulation reveals reorganized cortical outputs in amputees. Neurosci Lett 1990;116:379–386.

34 Brasil-Neto JP, Cohen LG, Pascual-Leone A, Jabir FK, Wall RT, Hallett M: Rapid reversible modulation of human motor outputs after transient deafferentation of the forearm: A study with transcranial magnetic stimulation. Neurology 1992;42:1302–1306.

35 Kucera P, Wiesendanger M: Do ipsilateral corticospinal fibers participate in the functional recovery following unilateral pyramidal lesions in monkeys? Brain Res 1985;348:297–303.

36 Cohen LG, Roth BJ, Wassermann EM, Topka H, Fuhr P, Schultz J, Hallett M: Magnetic stimulation of the human cerebral cortex, an indicator of reorganization in motor pathways in certain pathological conditions. J Clin Neurophysiol 1991;8:56–65.

37 Jenny AB: Commissural projections of the cortical hand motor area in monkeys. J Comp Neurol 1979;188: 137–146.

38 Rothwell JC, Day BL, Thompson PD, Marsden CD: Interruption of motor programmes by electrical or magnetic brain stimulation in man. Prog Brain Res 1989;80:467–472.

39 Müri RM, Hess CW, Meienberg O: Transcranial stimulation of the human frontal eye field by magnetic pulses. Exp Brain Res 1991;86:219–223.

40 Müri RM, Rösler KM, Hess CW: Influence of transcranial magnetic stimulation on the execution of memorised sequences of saccades in man. Exp Brain Res 1994;101:521–524.

41 Müri RM, Gaymard B, Rivaud S, Vermersch AI, Cassarini JF, Hess CW, Pierrot-Deseilligny C: Transcranial magnetic stimulation of the left posterior parietal and prefrontal cortex during memory-guided saccades. Is there a hemisphere asymmetry in saccade control? (Abstract) Congress of International Society for Neuroscience, Washington, Nov 1996.

42 Pascual-Leone A, Hallett M: Induction of errors in a delayed response task by repetitive transcranial magnetic stimulation of the dorsolateral prefrontal cortex. Neuroreport 1994;5:2517–2520.

Dr. Christian W. Hess, University Deparment of Neurology,
Inselspital Bern, CH–3010 Bern (Switzerland)

Hepp-Reymond M-C, Marini G (eds): Perspectives of Motor Behavior and Its Neural Basis.
Basel, Karger, 1997, pp 103–134

··········

Paths of Discovery in Human Motor Control

A Short Historical Perspective

Mario Wiesendanger[1]

Laboratory of Motor Systems, Department of Neurology, University of Bern,
Switzerland

Human motor control is a relatively young but thriving discipline. What might be
the reason for this extraordinary progress in human motor control? There are probably a
number of them, the strongest being our curiosity about how we, as human beings, move.
Although animals may move faster, often more elegantly, we also believe that, with the
emergence of man, capable to stand and move about upright with hands free to manipulate
skillfully, to communicate verbally, and to plan actions into the future, human motricity
has acquired new dimensions. These considerations have been particularly motivating for
studies of the special problem of balance control, imposed by the upright stance and gait,
the delicate hand function, and the important cognitive aspects of movement planning.
Through insight, human motricity is more anticipating, dependent on motor memory and
inner 'drives' (self-initiation), less stimulus-bound. Noninvasive methods which provide
more global and indirect hints on neural activity changes during motor performances are
booming: brain imaging studies with positron emission tomography (PET) or functional
magnetic resonance imaging (MRI), and also electroencephalographic (EEG) or magneto-
encephalographic (MEG) investigations all provide functional correlates of localized
changes of brain activity induced with motor behavior.

Human motor control has been nurtured by three traditional disciplines: physiology,
clinical neurology, and psychology. Although I organize my essay along these disciplines,
it appears that many concepts, originating in one discipline, soon found their way in other
disciplines. For example, the psychological concept of preparation for action was well
integrated in the work of the physiologist Hess and the neurologist Jung. Going through
the literature on human motor control, I realized that many of today's concepts in human
motricity have their roots in studies done early in this century. Also, I realized that there
are many significant contributions in the German literature which are not well known,
even among the German-speaking scientific community. Therefore, the aim of the present
chapter is to trace back some selected key issues in human motor control, to examine
from which discipline they originated and how they relate to modern ideas and concepts
of motor control.

[1] I thank Jean Massion and Marcus Jacobson for helpful comments and discussion. My research
is financially supported by the Swiss National Science Foundation.

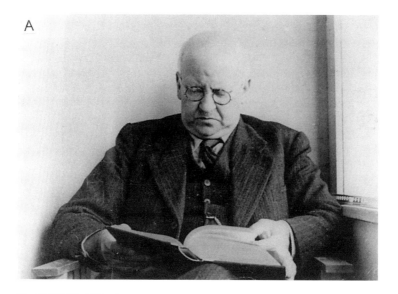

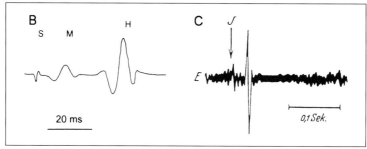

Fig. 1. A Portrait of Paul Hoffmann. **B** Reproduction of Hoffmann's first publication, 1910 [3], on the electrically elicited ankle reflex recorded electromyographically with high temporal resolution. From calculation of conduction times he deduced that the reflex is a two-neuron arc with only one synapse. S = Stimulus, M = direct excitation of the soleus muscle, H = reflex response. **C** First demonstration of the 'silent period' following the reflex response recorded on a background of voluntary activity. J = Stimulus application (the M response is minimal).

The Physiology Tradition

Reflexes, Tone and Motor Preparedness

For his time, Paul Hoffmann (1884–1962), a German physiologist in Freiburg (fig. 1A), was a rare exception in having performed most of his neurophysiological experiments in human subjects (his alternative were invertebrates). He is well known, also in the English-speaking scientific community, for his Reflex Studies [1], notably on what he called the 'Eigenreflex', now termed in his honor the H-reflex. He was first to claim that it is a monosynaptic two-neuron arc because the afferent and efferent conduction times made up just about the reflex latency, leaving no time for additional synapses. What makes the reflex still so important today was Hoffmann's further discovery that the reflex can be elicited electrically from the popliteal nerve (fig. 1B). This was the prerequisite for evoking the H-reflex with a constant afferent input, making it a reliable tool for exploring excitability of the motoneuron pool. Finally, he discovered the silent period in the muscle activity which follows the reflex compound potential and which was explained by inhibitory and disfacilitatory spinal mechanisms (fig. 1C). Hoffmann started reflex studies while he was a young assistant of Piper in Würzburg. To Piper [2] comes the merit of having introduced electromyography (EMG) in Germany. Following Piper, Hoffmann did all his studies with surface electrodes and, for a long time, with string galvanometers. He was intrigued by this technique, realizing that it provided an indirect means of monitoring the central commands. The first results were published in 1910 [3], but outside Germany the work of Hoffmann and his pupils began to be appreciated only after World War II. Neither in the famous monograph on reflexes from the school of Sherrington [4], nor in the monograph on 'Discovery of Reflexes' by Liddell [5], is there any mention of Hoffmann's work. According to Jung [6], Sherrington knew about it, but was skeptical about the monosynaptic nature of the phasic stretch reflex as claimed by Hoffmann; but direct proof arrived in 1943 with the cat experiments of Lloyd [7]. It was with the publications of Magladery and McDougal [8] at Johns Hopkins, and of Paillard [9] at the Collège de France that the H-reflex area was opened, flourishing up to the present day. Both groups made intensive use of the H-reflex technology and started the now classical assessment of excitability changes by means of the H-reflex size which is modulated by a preceding conditioning stimulus. Magladery [10] also proved the monosynaptic nature of the H-reflex in humans by directly stimulating the dorsal root and recording the response from the ventral root. Until the present time, the H-reflex has been a very useful tool to address two questions: First, can specific spinal circuits be singled out in the human spinal cord? An early H-reflex study in this direction concerned the Ia-inhibitory circuit [11]; further studies followed on the Renshaw, Ib, and presynaptic inhibitory circuits [12–15]. These proved important avenues for assessing quantitatively the involvement of specific spinal pathways in central motor disorders. Second, how is the motoneuron pool modulated in excitability during the perfor- mance of voluntary movements? It was first shown by Gurfinkel et al. [16; see also 17, 18] that the H-reflex, used as a probing test response, was facilitated well before EMG onset of a rapid voluntary movement. More recently, by means of H-reflex testing, a number of studies have examined the underlying mechanisms of task-dependent excitability changes in the spinal cord [14, 19, 20]. One important outcome was that the reflex gain is variable and adjusted to the actual movement 'program' [21].

Muscle tone and posture were key issues in the laboratory of Sherrington who exploited extensively the decerebrate cat model which, as he well recognized, is only a caricature of posture, normally checked by the higher motor centers. The Sherrington school considered posture, and its underlying muscle tone, to be reflex in nature [22]. The main arguments were (a) that decerebrate rigidity vanished after dorsal rhizotomy, and (b) that postural adaptations can easily be obtained by proprioceptive and vestibular activation procedures. These were the tonic labyrinthine and neck reflexes, investigated in detail by Magnus [23] and Rademaker [24]. These were important observations relating to the reactive mode of postural adjustments. However, the very nature of reduced animal preparations precluded the manifestation of the anticipatory (or proactive) generation of postural tone. It is now evident that the latter proactive mode is at least as important, if not more, than the reactive reflex component.

The story on human posture started with simple considerations and also simple experiments. The physical necessity of anticipation was already recognized by Leonardo da Vinci (cited in Gahéry [25]): '... when a man stands motionless upon his feet and then

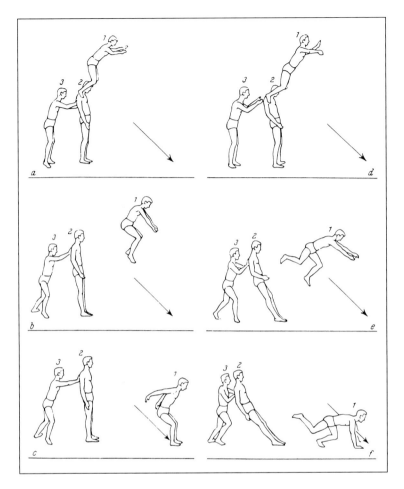

Fig. 2. Model of a goal-directed action redrawn from a motion picture taken by Hess (1943; cf. Akert, 1981 [26]). Student 1 performs the goal-directed movement, student 2 represents the postural support, and student 3 is the 'tone-setter'. In a–c, the goal-directed leap is successful because there is an adequate postural support. In d–f, however, the leap misses the goal because of an unprepared readiness for support; an emerging reactive support is too late for proper movement execution. Drawing reproduced from Jung [120].

extends his arm in front of his chest, he must move backwards a natural weight equal to that … which he moves towards the front.'

Walter Rudolf Hess (1881–1973), Professor of Physiology in Zürich and a brilliant experimenter with an integrative view on physiology, devised with much ingenuity a human model of posture to demonstrate the need of a parallel control of movement and posture to his students. This was documented in a movie [see 26, p. 266]. The drawings of figure 2 were made after this movie, and this figure later used by Jung [27], who had been a visiting scientist in the Hess laboratory in Zürich, for illustrating the point of postural anticipation in the Handbook of the American Physiological Society [28]. It should be recalled that Hess had been a pioneer in working in chronically prepared cats. With low-intensity

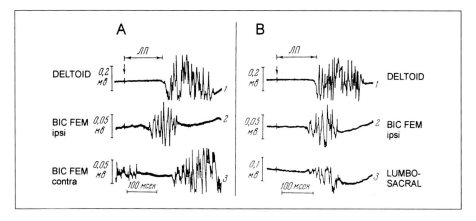

Fig. 3. First demonstration of anticipatory postural adjustment in self-motion (arm elevation, deltoid EMG burst). Note that excitation (ipsilateral biceps femoris, lumbosacral) or suppression (contralateral biceps femoris) precede the goal-directed arm movement. **A** and **B** are from two experiments. Reproduced from Belenki et al. [29].

electrical stimulation within the diencephalon and the brainstem, he was able to elicit or modify natural motor behavior [26]. Especially when stimulating the midbrain tegmentum, he could appreciate how eyes, head and trunk are orchestrated for a unified, purposeful and goal-directed action: he was convinced that the postural components were centrally integrated and not reflex actions.

It was only in 1967 that Belenki et al. [29] published their seminal paper, proving with EMG recordings that postural adaptations in the case of self-motion occur simultaneously or even before intended movements. These Russian scientists, coming from the Bernstein tradition of human movement control, used (knowingly?) exactly the arm-elevation paradigm Leonardo da Vinci was contemplating about (see citation above). It became clear to the authors that this was a dynamic and complex stabilizing synergy which could be recorded in many muscles of the trunk and the lower limbs in conjunction with, not as reaction to, the aiming arm movement (fig. 3). The impact of this paper was considerable, and research in postural adjustments and stabilization has much advanced our knowledge in this field during the last 20 years [e.g. 30, 31].

In an opening address to a posture symposium, Granit [32] also commented on tone, not as a reflex phenomenon, but as a preparatory device preceding movements. This is '... *a concept of tone as a state ...*', or '*a kind of state of light excitation*', leading to '*motor preparedness*'. Much recent experimental work on muscle tone and posture deals with its neuronal organization and significance in motricity. 'Tonogenic' centers in the brainstem with their descending, widely and bilaterally distributed axons were studied by Mori et al. [33]. Reticulospinal fiber systems, together with descending serotonergic and noradrenergic fibers [34, 35] are likely to play a role in what Granit called 'motor preparedness', i.e. a postural state rather than a phasic postural adjustment. In behaving monkeys performing a choice reaction paradigm, tonic increases or decreases of EMG in shoulder muscles were observed during a noncued waiting period while the monkey expected the occurrence of one or the other 'go' signal [36, 37]. Parallel increases of tonic activity of neurons in the primary and secondary motor cortical areas were also frequently seen during the waiting period, i.e. before the monkeys obtained the cue for response selection. We therefore suggested that this tonic activity might be the neural correlate of postural preparedness. In monkeys trained to perform an arm flexion task, Mellah et al. [38] discovered activity of small motor units with a low recruitment threshold which started to discharge at the beginning of the preparatory phase, with activity progressively increasing and abruptly stopping at movement onset. Fifteen percent of the recorded motor units fell into this category whereas the majority of motor units were related to movement execution, fired phasically and were of the high-threshold type.

Kurt Wachholder: Coordination of Volitional Posture and Movements

As EMG techniques became available, a window was opened for looking into the working of the spinal cord. The physiologist was first to exploit EMG for a systematic investigation of posture and limb movements in healthy human subjects and who provided the first account on some principles in human coordination. When Wachholder (1893–1961) started his brilliant series of experiments in humans, he had already been confronted with the problem of coordination from his dissertation on the spinal frog ('Über den Wischreflex des Frosches', University of Bonn, 1920). After moving to the Physiology Institute at the University of Breslau, Wachholder published within 4 years 11 papers in *Pflügers Archiv*, partly together with Altenburger (the latter, together with Foerster, was to play an important role in introducing EMG into clinical neurology, as detailed below). This series of papers was the substance of an extensive review published by Wachholder [39] in 1928 which contains most of the data of the original publications and to which I mainly refer. A novel and decisive step was Wachholder's use of two and most sensitive string galvanometers for simultaneous recording of the activity from a pair of muscles. Together with the two EMG traces he also recorded, with a high-speed kymograph camera, angular position of monoarticular movements and the time signal. Finally, he was also the first to record EMG activity with the more specific intramuscular needle electrodes. Altogether this meant a remarkable technical improvement, made possible by financial support from the Rockefeller Foundation. At the age of 35 years, he wrote his habilitation thesis on the coordination of voluntary movements and was promoted as Professor of Physiology. His work on coordination of human voluntary movements was essentially completed in 1928. When he was appointed as Chairman of Physiology in Rostock in 1933 (fig. 4), he started to work on a number of different nonneurophysiological subjects, such as metabolism and nutrition. Not being a member of the party, he had to face all the odds of the Nazi time and to lead the institute through the disastrous war time. New difficulties arose some years after the war with the new Stalinistic regime heavily interfering with the University affairs. Fed up with the situation, he decided in 1953 to 'emigrate' to Bonn ('Republikflucht'!), accepting the Chair of Physiology from his former teacher Verworn[2].

What were Wachholder's major conceptual contributions in human motor control? As indicated by the titles of his doctoral and habilitation theses, his research was focused on the issue of movement coordination. His 'Leitmotiv' is that physiological investigations of voluntary movements can only be successful if the (mental) project of the movement ('Bewegungsentwurf'), i.e. the aim, is taken into account as an integral component of the

---

[2] I follow here a manuscript of a biographical note by J. Burmeister who was a former member of the Physiology Institute in Rostock. The manuscript is intended for publication in 'Biographisches Lexikon für Mecklenburg', Schmidt-Röhmhild Verlag, Lübeck, Germany, and was kindly sent to me by the present Chairman of Physiology in Rostock, Prof. C. Pfeiffer.

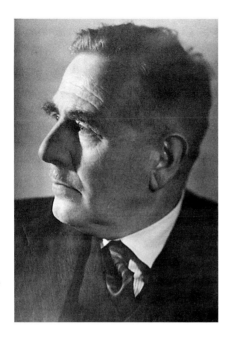

Fig. 4. Portrait of K. Wachholder (photograph from the Institute of Physiology in Rostock, Germany).

study. Volition is centered around the goal, not around the details of the movement paths; the control of the latter is to a large extent automatic and not a conscious process. Reflexes and even passive properties of the muscles, in short all components which make up the movement, are bound together for a unitary action dictated by the goal. That means that the various factors must covary for goal achievement. Some of these thoughts were not new at the time. For example, Kohnstamm [40] already defined coordination in 1901 as the principle of constraining muscles to a spatial-temporal activation pattern for common goal achievement. Similarly, Foerster [41] defined coordination as the capacity of the organism to use muscles for a unitary purposeful action. These central ideas in motor control now began to penetrate actual research, including that of Bernstein in Moscow and also that of Hess in Zürich.

New in the approach of Wachholder was his experimental design to investigate quantitatively the rules which make up the unitary goal. He started from the premise that there is no pre-established scheme ('program') for the rich repertoire of movements, and that it would be hopeless to find specific rules for each action. He deliberately varied the constraints in his investigation of relatively simple movements, for example the effects of loads or instructions, such as the speed of the forthcoming movement. The research plan was to investigate how these independent variables, i.e. external or internal constraints, affect movement execution. The measurements of the dependent variables (mostly temporal) should then reveal the rules that govern coordination.

This is well described in the introductory chapter of Wachholder's review published in 'Ergebnisse der Physiologie' in 1928 [39]. The monograph is truly a find abounding with discoveries on coordination of voluntary movements. Fessard, at the Collège de France in Paris, was first, outside Germany, to realize the importance of Wachholder's work and he dedicated one of his first papers to it ('Le Mouvement Volontaire, d'après K. Wachholder') [42, 43]. Later, his own experimental work was inspired by Wachholder's concept that coordination is conditional on the movement project [44, 45]. As a research associate of Fessard, Paillard incorporated these concepts in his excellent chapter on 'The Patterning of Skilled Movements' [46], published in the Handbook of Physiology of the American Physiological Society, with due mention of the pioneering work of Wachholder and Altenburger. Paillard's early work with Fessard, performed at the Institut Marey in Paris, was clearly influenced by Wachholder's concepts of coordination.

Wachholder's recordings were technically speaking the best and clearest at the time. Only a few issues, which I find still of interest today, will be shortly discussed and illustrated in figures 5–7. He demonstrates how posture (defined as a position of the limb when active and passive torques are in equilibrium) is an integral part of intention: movements are transitions from one equilibrium position to another. Posture adapts according to the set ('Einstellung') and to the external conditions; in this sense, posture is always a compensation. For example, posture is differently organized depending on whether the subject intends to maintain position or force. He recognized the importance of the 'passive' properties of the muscle and the surrounding tissue for generating restoring forces (not accompanied by action potentials) which he measured by loading the moving part at the reversal points for anulling the rebound. He furthermore showed how intentional stiffening enhanced the elastic restoring property of the muscle when posture was perturbed, or that the length-tension properties of the muscle allow for independent control of length and tension, at least in a limited range. This explains for example how the hand can be passively displaced without the generation of any active tension (as revealed by the silent EMG), provided the displacement is not too large or too rapid.

Turning to movements, he wisely chose relatively simple situations. Thus he simplified the problem by avoiding gravity with adequate support and supination of the forearm when studying wrist flexions and extensions. By limiting the movement to the wrist, he also avoided the complication of interaction torques of distant limb segments. He then systematically studied these movements by playing with the independent variables of stiffening, speed, amplitude, and imposed weight, analyzing the dependent EMG variables of the main agonist-antagonist muscle pair and trajectories. Here are some of his remarkable observations: a slow movement executed without any additional stiffening ('lockere Bewegung') is characterized by low agonist EMG activity with action potentials firing at about 10 Hz during the whole course of the movement, without any activity in the antagonist (fig. 5A). As the movement is executed a bit faster (fig. 5B), the agonist activity becomes more prominent, but often ends, or is considerably diminished before the new target is attained because sufficient moment of inertia brings the hand to the target. A weak burst in the antagonist comes in with some delay. With still faster movements (fig. 5C), the antagonist movement occurs earlier. The significance of the delayed antagonist activity was seen in terms of a braking function, today a generally accepted notion; the earlier onset with fast movements is explicable by the need to compensate for the larger momentum of the hand. When comparing intended movements of large and small amplitudes, but of equal velocity, the antagonist burst comes in earlier with small movement amplitudes, again suggesting its role for braking automatically the movement at the proper time for goal achievement. With very fast movements, the antagonistic burst appeared with a delay as short as 10 ms proving that it was not a stretch reflex produced by the hand displacement, but rather a centrally programmed and integral part of the intended motor task. This was further substantiated by blocking the afferents of the antagonist with novocain which did not abolish the antagonist burst as it would were it a reflex.

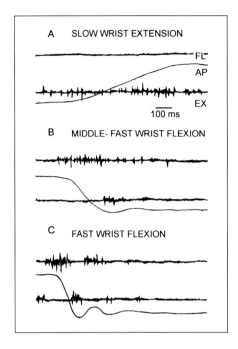

Fig. 5. EMG patterns of antagonistic muscle pair (wrist flexors and extensors). Subject was requested to perform successively faster movements (**A–C**). Note reciprocal pattern in the faster movements (see also text for further details). Redrawn from Wachholder [39].

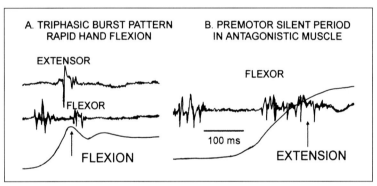

Fig. 6. First documentation of reciprocal 3-phasic burst pattern and of premovement silent period in antagonistic muscle. Redrawn from Wachholder [39].

Wachholder is best rememberd for the by now classic 3-burst pattern of simple ballistic movements (fig. 6A). Forty years later, we rediscovered and published the same observation of a 3-burst pattern duly citing Wachholder [47]. But this paper, published in German in the *Schweizer Archiv für Neurologie und Psychiatrie*, went unnoticed; it was the paper of Angel [48], i.e. 50 years after Wachholder, which led to an explosion of further research on the 3-burst pattern [e.g. 49–54]. It eventually also led to the pulse-height control hypothesis of Ghez [55]. It is not the place here to go into the details of some controversies; the main conclusions of Wachholder still stand and the lively pursuit of research of Wachholder's discovery only emphasizes its importance for understanding some basic principles of voluntary movements.

Associated with this line of research was the observation of Wachholder [39] that, before the antagonist comes in, pre-existing hold activity is inhibited (fig. 6B). This premotion silent period was further stressing the central nature of agonist-antagonist patterning. The phenomenon was also rediscovered much later by Hufschmidt and Hufschmidt [56] and continues to raise interest [50, 57–59]. A further line of continued research [e.g. 60] was Wachholder's discovery of distinct functional muscle compartments [39].

Rhythm Generation

Rhythms are common in motor behavior. Not only are locomotion, breathing and mastication rhythmic, but also many voluntary manual performances. As remarked by Wachholder [39], rhythmic movements are the most economical ones because passive restoring forces are best exploited in cyclic movements (economy was an important consideration in the physiological work of Wachholder). Accordingly, he investigated with particular care the reciprocal and exactly timed pattern of the agonist and antagonist EMG traces when rhythmic flexion-extension movements of the wrist were performed at different speeds. This is shown in his summarizing diagram of figure 7B.

From the first EMG recordings of voluntary activity, Piper [2] concluded that the muscle 'action currents' occur rhythmically at a relatively fixed frequency of 50 Hz. But with more selective intramuscular electrodes and improved amplification, Wachholder found that the single action currents varied between 5 and 75 Hz. Although Wachholder seemed to ignore the concept of motor units (the term was introduced in 1925 by Liddell and Sherrington [61]), it seems likely that Wachholder's 'single action currents' were in fact discharges of single motor units. He noted that the frequency of these potentials rarely exceeded 50 Hz and then only for short periods and with stronger contractions (these were obviously the larger potentials of the phasic motor units recruited at higher threshold). For sustained activity, the dominating frequency was found to be more typically around 10 Hz. He clearly distinguished 'rhythms' of single action currents (i.e. single motor units) from the rhythm of grouped discharges of several action currents which were separated by periods of silence or strongly reduced activity. He was obviously intrigued by this population phenomenon because he illustrated and discussed it on several occasions in his review. He found that some subjects have a pronounced rhythm, others less or not at all and that it occurs during holding as well as during moving (see slow movement in figure 7A). It is provoked regularly if a very strong contraction has to be maintained over a prolonged time, i.e. when the muscle fatigues. In this case a disturbing fatigue tremor is clearly visible. But what is the functional significance of the normal 10-Hz rhythm occurring with moderate contractions? Because of the low-pass filter properties of the muscle, one can normally see only a minimal physiological tremor, i.e. small undulations in the position trace (fig. 7A). Wachholder does not address the issue of functional significance, except to say that the slight departure from complete smoothness in the contractions of unfatigued muscles was hardly a disturbing factor. In one respect, however oscillation around 10 Hz appears to be a useful mechanism for at least one purposeful performance as shown by Schlapp [62]: it is used by violin players for producing vibrato!

Later, the 10-Hz EMG rhythm was studied by a number of investigators. Lippold [63] came to the conclusion that it was an expression of an oscillation in the stretch reflex pathway. But this point remained controversial for a long time. Whereas Matthews and Muir [64] and Burne et al. [65] agreed with the stretch reflex hypothesis, others advanced arguments against it [66, 67]. Hagbarth and Young [68] proved by microneuronography that muscle spindles were indeed rhythmically active and suggested that the stretch reflex

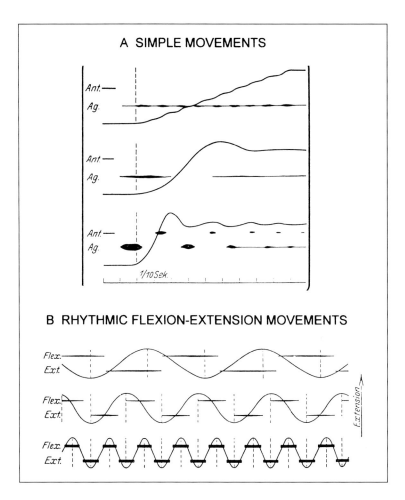

Fig. 7. A Schematic representation of innervation pattern of subjects performing simple hand movements at different speeds. See 10 Hz undulation of position trace in the slow movement. Reciprocal interactions with the antagonist EMG (black) in fast movements. From Wachholder (1930). **B** Reciprocal innervation pattern in rhythmic flexion-extension movements of the hand. From Wachholder [39].

could enhance (but not cause) the tremor. Most recently, Vallbo and Wessberg [69] made a careful analysis of the 10-Hz rhythm of long finger muscles occurring most clearly during slow finger movements. They showed that with faster movements the rhythmic angular velocity peaks increased, however without change in frequency. Wessberg et al. [70] also confirmed Hagbarth and Young [68] that spindles were indeed discharging in bursts at 10 Hz, concluding that these discharges were modulated in response to the tremor, rather than causing the EMG rhythm. Thus, the conclusions of the Swedish authors and of Wachholder were similar, notably that the origin is central. The former went even further, suggesting that the rhythmic EMG was the result of a pulsatile descending command signal [70]. This highly interesting proposition remains to be proven.

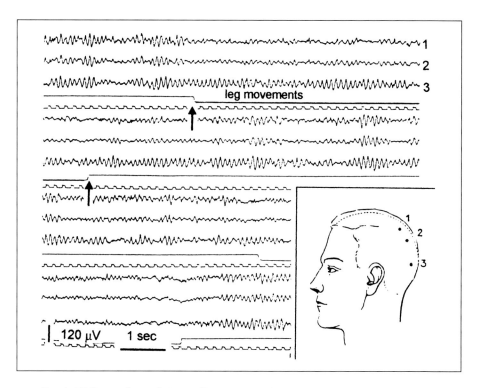

Fig. 8. EEG recordings of Kornmüller [74], showing desynchronization and occurrence of β-activity during leg movements. These EEG changes were restricted to the central leg representation at the electrode positions 1 and 2.

There is currently a strong interest in rhythmicity of neuronal populations at the cortical level because it is felt that oscillations, as a population phenomenon, may be an important organizing principle used by the brain to create dynamic spatiotemporal coherence patterns necessary for coordination [see e.g. 71, 72]. It is not clear in which structures the EEG rhythms are generated. Candidates are intrinsic pacemakers in the cortex, or extracortical thalamic and olivocerebellar generators [73]. That EEG rhythms may somehow be related with the production of movements was already shown in the first EEG recordings of Berger. A good example is taken from recordings made in 1940 by Kornmüller [74] who worked, in competition with Berger, at the Brain Research Institute in Berlin. Figure 12 shows how a leg movement produced a desynchronization of the EEG. This was most marked in leads overlying the leg representation (traces 1 and 2 in figure 8), without an effect in the more distant visual cortex (trace 3). Similar observations were performed by Jasper and Penfield [75] in 1949 at the Montreal Neurological Institute. In recent years, Pfurtscheller and co-workers [76, 77] have done extensive series of experiments on these localized desynchronizations which could be mapped in the sensorimotor cortex. Of particular interest was the demonstration that desynchronization actually started about 1.7 s before movement onset. Furthermore, Pfurtscheller et al. [78] discovered that, embedded in the periods of desynchronization, short epochs of 40 Hz could occur around movement onset. Kristeva-Feige et al. [79] mapped narrow-band activity at about 19 Hz during an imposed waiting period before execution of the movement.

That the activity of pyramidal tract neurons is grouped together for rhythmic discharges around 10 Hz before and during intended movements, as suggested by Wessberg et al. [70], has not been observed in recordings from the motor cortex. However, oscillatory activity at the higher rates of 20–40 Hz has now been discovered in recordings from the motor cortex of monkeys performing skilled finger movements [80–82]. It is still unclear to what extent these phenomena are linked to the mental project of the movement, to general readiness to move, or to movement execution [83, 84].

The Neurology Tradition

In Germany, the methodology of nerve stimulation and EMG, pioneered by Hoffmann and his co-workers, was first exploited in neurology for examining peripheral neuromuscular disorders and not for exploring the central nervous system. It was as if Hoffmann made his discovery at the wrong time: in Germany, there was no other active physiology institute studying the central nervous system as for example in England. As pointed out by Jung [6], physiologists using electrophysiological tools for anything else than peripheral nerves or muscles were suspect! It was at this critical moment that the neurologist and neurosurgeon Otfried Foerster from Breslau took the lead in the electrophysiological exploration of central motor disorders.

Foerster, the Neurologist and Neurosurgeon

Foerster (1873–1941) was a neurophysiologically minded clinician who established himself as an internationally recognized neurologist [for a biographical sketch, see 85]. In view of the increasing number of gunshot wounds of the brain in World War I, he felt obliged to specialize also in neurosurgery (at a time when, on the continent, neurosurgery hardly existed as an own discipline). He was successful in surgical interventions on the brain and soon also pioneered the first successful operations on spinal tumors in Germany. Influenced by readings of Sherrington on the reflex nature of muscle tone, he was led to perform a series of dorsal rhizotomies in severely spastic patients. As expected from the results on deafferentation in decerebrate cats [86], spasticity in patients was abolished [87]. Unfortunately, the long-range outcome was not satisfactory for upper limb spasticity. Interestingly, this rather heroic procedure has been re-introduced with a more conservative interruption of sensory inflow. Attempts have been made to spare lemniscal fibers for cutaneous sensation, and to cut only the segment of the lateral and central rootlets, containing the small-diameter pain fibers as well as the large 'myotatic fibers' believed to subserve the myotatic reflex [88].

Besides his special interest in the spinal cord, Foerster was also much interested in the normal and abnormal function of the cortex. He soon gained a vast surgical experience in removing cortical tumors and resections of epileptic cortex. For example, in his extensive review on cortical motor areas, he described the consequences of 20 cases with localized excisions in the premotor cortex alone [89]. It is through this work that he began to use electrical stimulation to delimit the various subfields before surgical excisions.

Foerster established many international contacts. In England he met Sherrington and was invited to deliver the Hughlings Jackson Lecture [90]. He was also invited to the United States to act as a 'chief surgeon' at the renowned neurosurgery clinic of Cushing. Foerster also received many guests at his clinic in Breslau. Among them was Wilder Penfield who stayed at the Foerster clinic in 1928 and who is now well known for his extensive use of electrical stimulation of the human cortex during neurosurgical operations (see below). Finally, one has to mention Margareth Kennard (from the school of Fulton at Yale) who is best known for the 'Kennard principle' (higher plastic capacity of the immature brain). Kennard [91] later published an exhaustive chapter for the book 'The Precentral Motor Cortex'[3], reviewing the effects of motor cortex stimulations and ablations.

Foerster's Collaboration with Altenburger

Altenburger (1902–1938) who had assisted Wachholder in the EMG study of hand movements at the Physiology Institute in Breslau, was hired in 1925 by Foerster who urgently needed a physiologically trained assistant. This led to a fruitful collaboration during the next 10 years. Altenburger entered the academic career and became professor in the mid-30s. He wrote a monumental review on the entire field of electrophysiological applications in neurology for the Handbuch der Neurologie [92] which appeared in 1937, i.e. 1 year before his career ended abruptly when he died of cancer at the age of 36. The clinical research program was to exploit the technical know-how and the concepts of coordination developed by Wachholder and to make it available to Neurology. Thus a laboratory was installed in the basement of the clinic for research with the new EMG technology on patients with central movement disorders. It turned out that the results about the coordination of simple voluntary movements in these patients were not straight-forward: they varied a great deal and were sometimes undistinguishable from the normal pattern. In patients with a 'pyramidal syndrome', they found an increased tendency for rhythmic grouping in the EMG at about 10 Hz. In severe cases, they found that already in slow movements, the antagonist muscle is active during the whole movement; in faster movements, the antagonistic burst tended to come in very early, with both agonist and antagonist displaying a prolonged and rhythmic activity. The 3-burst pattern, typical of normal fast movements, is thus obscured in the protracted activity. However, the authors also note that similar patterns may be obtained in healthy subjects who cannot relax well. Patients with 'extrapyramidal' rigidity showed often persisting activity in the resting limb, with typical tremor bursts. Changes in the pattern of active movements with abnormal activity in the antagonist, loss of a clear 3-burst pattern, and the occurrence of action tremor were also documented. In cerebellar patients, they found disturbances of the 3-burst pattern, for example a lack of the antagonistic burst resulting in an overshoot, or the occurrence of intention tremor.

The major emphasis of their investigations was, however, on reflex testing and the attempt to correlate spasticity or rigidity with the stretch reflex response. It appears that Foerster was caught in the Sherringtonian concept of reflex nature of muscle tone and posture. For him, as for other renowned neurologists at the time [e.g. 93], a decerebrate cat was considered a proper animal model for human spasticity. Today, most would agree that it is not, neither for spasticity nor for parkinsonian rigidity. The other problem was that quantification of the response was hardly possible since averaging procedures with smoothing, rectification and integration of the EMG were not available. It thus appears that the gain of these pioneering

---

[3] This was a landmark publication dealing with the motor cortex and its pyramidal tract outflow. It reflects very well the state of the art at that time, and from an American perspective. It is remarkable that this book, published in the middle of the war with Germany, was dedicated to Otfried Foerster 'who stimulated the recent renaissance of interest in the activity of the human cerebral cortex, emphasized the correlation of its physiological activity with its microscopic structure, recognized the importance of animal experimentation for the understanding of human problems, insisted on the confirmation of the results of animal experimentation by observations on man.'

clinical studies was relatively modest. According to Jung [6], physiologists hardly took notice of the work of Altenburger and Foerster, except Hoffmann who got into polemics with Foerster about his interpretation of the stretch reflex.

I believe there is a lesson for today: For too long the study of central motor disorders was focused on what Evarts called 'laboratory reflexes' [94], and too little on mechanisms of whole actions (which may include reflex components). Instead of testing 'laboratory reflexes' in the traditional way, one needs to adopt the perturbation paradigm in the context of 'everyday' tasks; for example, testing spastic subjects when they have to grasp a manipulandum and to hold it with changing predictive and unpredictive loads, as it may occur in the real world when, on a walk with a dog on the leash, the dog suddenly chases a cat.

Foerster's Contacts with the Vogts

Cécile Vogt (1875–1962) and Oskar Vogt (1870–1955), well known for their cyto- and myeloarchitectonic studies on the cerebral cortex, thalamus and the basal ganglia, as well as for their parallel electrical stimulation studies on the cerebral cortex, established themselves in Berlin as the leading experts in brain research. This is remarkable because they succeeded without being in a traditional university institute of anatomy or physiology; instead they were founders of probably the first interdisciplinary institute devoted to brain research. With the name of this institution – 'Neurobiologisches Laboratorium' – they also introduced the now current term of neurobiology. In 1930, the Vogts inaugurated a new spacious Hirnforschungsinstitut in Berlin-Dahlem which was generously cofinanced by the Rockefeller Foundation and the Kaiser-Wilhelm Gesellschaft (the predecessor of the Max-Planck-Gesellschaft). With its modern equipment and its various methodological disciplines, including also a small neurology clinic, it was unique in the world. Its sad fate starting before World War II, and its end in 1945, is another story [for the interested reader, see 95–97].

Foerster's interest in the Vogts was evident: they had established the maps of the cerebral cortex in a number of subhuman primates. Of particular interest for Foerster was that the cartography relied not only on cytoarchitectonic criteria, but also on electrical stimulation mapping. The Vogts claimed to have obtained a perfect match between the two maps (fig. 9, from Vogt and Vogt [98]). Although one has to admit that this cannot be ascertained on the basis of the published material, and also that their 'hairsharp' areal bounderies were often contested by experts of cytoarchitectonic mapping, it provided a basis for Foerster to embark on numerous explorations with electrical stimulation of the brain surface during neurosurgical interventions. Synthesizing the individual results in one map, Foerster [89, 90] obtained a remarkable resemblance with a 'constructed' map of the Vogts who had simply transferred their monkey data to a human brain by 'homologizing' the various areas of the two species! This was their 'human homolog' [98]. Both, the Vogts in the monkey brain and Foerster in the human brain, described a separate motor field on the mesial side of the hemisphere, in front of the foot representation, from which complex adversive movements of the trunk, forelimb, head and eyes were elicited by repetitive and rather strong surface stimuli. This was the discovery of what Penfield later termed the 'supplementary motor area' (see below). Wilder Penfield learned from this early work when he came to the Foerster clinic in 1928; important for Penfield's later career were also the many opportunities to participate in Foerster's neurosurgical interventions, combined with brain stimulation, aiming at localizing epileptic foci for precise and minimal surgical removal of pathologic brain tissue and scars [99].

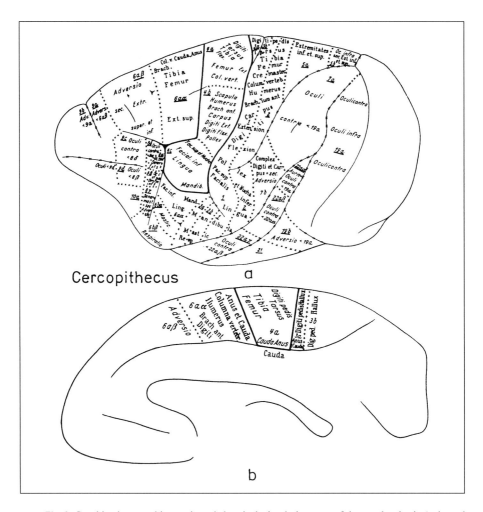

Fig. 9. Combined cytoarchitectonic and electrical stimulation map of the monkey brain (**a**, lateral and **b**, mesial surfaces). The motor cortex is divided into a primary field (4a, 4b, 4c), a secondary field (6aα), and a tertiary field (6aβ). Isolated movements are elicited with lowest intensity from the primary motor field, more complex movements are observed when stimulating at higher intensity in areas 6aα and 6aβ. Characteristic adversive synergies of the eyes, head and trunk can be evoked by stimulation of the field 6ab ('Adversio'). The 'adversive field' on the mesial hemisphere was later termed 'supplementary motor area' by Penfield. Note that motor effects, particulary eye movements, may also be elicited by stimulation of areas posterior to the central sulcus. From Vogt and Vogt [98].

Foerster had another link with the Vogts: he had been called to Moscow in 1922 as a leading neurologist for treating Lenin who suffered from a stroke with a right-sided hemiplegia and aphasia; he stayed there until Lenin's death in 1924. At this point, Oskar Vogt was called to Moscow to study Lenin's brain. To this end, a new Brain Research Institute was built according to the recommendations of Oskar Vogt. After 5 years of studies, he found that Lenin's cortex had unusually large pyramids of layer III in the intact hemisphere, and he ventured to state that this was an expression of Lenin's genius. In

1928, Penfield went with Foerster to visit the Vogt Institute in Berlin where Oskar Vogt showed them the histological sections with the giant cortical cells of Lenin. Penfield recounts his more than skeptic feelings about this visit in his memoirs 'No Man Alone – A Neurosurgeon's Life', an episode which was recently republished by Kreutzberg et al. [95].

As is well known, this line of functional neurosurgery of the cerebral cortex with the help of electrical stimulation was extensively continued by Penfield and Jasper at the Montreal Neurological Institute. After a detailed investigation of the mesial frontal cortex, Penfield and Jasper [100] changed the name of 'mesial adversive field' of the Vogts to 'supplementary motor area', or briefly SMA. In Europe, explorations of the human SMA were resumed in 1966 by Talairach and Bancaud [101]. They used implants of electrode arrays which were oriented horizontally from the external surface to the inner surface of the dorsal-most part of the frontal cortex. By leaving the leads in situ during several days, they were able to stimulate and to record brain activity in various motor areas, including the SMA and the anterior cingulate area. This was done before the surgical intervention in order to precisely localize the epileptic foci and to delimit areal boundaries. The patients were awake and able to talk and move. Since the late 70s, a large amount of research on the SMA of monkeys and human subjects, including neurological patients, has been published which is of great importance for the entire issue of motor control. It is not the place to review this burgeoning field of research except to say that it made people aware of the great importance of cognitive aspects of motor control which have much to do with the 'movement project', and also with the concept of division of labor in subareas of the motor cortex in the wide sense. Many of the recent findings concerning the functional role of the SMA in humans were made possible by the advent of brain mapping techniques with EEG or MEG, PET and functional MRI. Although we are still far from understanding the detailed role(s) of the SMA in the organization of voluntary movements, it seems clear that its function goes beyond the original 'supplementary', i.e. auxiliary connotation [for a recent account on research and clinical findings on the SMA, see 102–104].

The Psychology Tradition

The Reaction Time Paradigm
Donders [105] introduced this paradigm as a research tool in experimental psychology, and the physiologist Exner [106] defined reaction time as the elapsed time between presentation of a motivating stimulus ('Motivreiz') and the ensuing movement. The founders of psychophysics (von Frey, Weber and Fechner) were more interested in sensation and perception. Wundt, who directed the first Institute of Experimental Psychology in Germany, had a particular interest in the timing of perceptive awareness. For example, Kraepelin [107] who later became a renowned psychiatrist spent a short time in Wundt's laboratory, attempting to measure mental reactions with Hipp's chronoscope and the changes produced by 'poisons' (small amounts of ether, chloroform, coffee, alcohol, morphium). It was only at the beginning of the 20th century that movement studies began to influence concepts in motor control. Külpe, a former assistant of Wundt, together with the psychologists Ach and Watt in Würzburg introduced, not without opposition from Wundt, the concept of 'Einstellung' (=set) in the context of motricity [108–110]. In 1922, Helena Vörckel [111], who worked at the Wundt Institute in Leipzig, was first to introduce EMG assessment of reaction times. It appears that all major issues that can be studied with the reaction time paradigm had already been approached by the first quarter of the 20th century. In 1927,

Wirth [112] wrote an amazingly comprehensive review chapter for the Handbuch der Normalen und Pathologischen Physiologie. In it, he discusses (1) the influence of set, alertness, attention, motivation; (2) the role of modality and intensity of the imperative stimulus; (3) the degree of perceptual recognition or discrimination; (4) the effects of a preceding warning stimulus, regularity of stimulus presentation, predictive versus unpredictive stimulus presentation; (5) the effects of posture and motor set; (6) the number of choices involved in the task; (7) the influence of neuropharmacological substances, and (8) the effect of brain lesions.

Reaction time studies have been for a long time an almost exclusive prerogative of psychologists. For example, the contributors to a relatively recent book on reaction time, edited by Welford [113] in 1980, were all psychologists. To them comes also the credit of having exploited this paradigm to capture the rules underlying sensorimotor processing and to establish models [114]. Some models advocate a discrete serial stage processing, others parallel processing. This issue, being of general interest for understanding motor control, has been much debated by motor physiologists interested also in the subserving anatomical pathways and relays. Glickstein [115] addressed the question at an early stage and suggested, on the basis of electrophysiologically recorded sensory responses and electrical stimulations, that the observed visuomotor reaction times in monkeys are not compatible with a 'simple series-wired interpretation of reaction-time'. The consensus today would probably be that the two modes of processing, serial and parallel, coexist.

It took a long time until physiologists and neurologists recognized the great value of the reaction time paradigm. We assessed reaction times in healthy subjects and in parkinsonian patients who, at that time, were not yet under DOPA medication [47]. In both groups, simple and visual choice reaction time was measured (fig. 10). In controls, the choice reaction time was on average 75% longer than the simple reaction time. Only choice but not simple reaction time increased significantly with age. In parkinsonian we noted, as Altenburger and Foerster before, the often disturbed 3-burst pattern with prolonged non-reciprocal movement-related activity (in 2 patients with grouped discharges as an expression of action tremor). In spite of the massive alteration in coordination, the simple reaction times were in the normal range. Surprisingly, choice reaction time was mostly in the normal range, except in 1 patient who had a massive prolongation of her choice reaction time (with a normal simple reaction time). Interestingly, this was the only patient who had also a very marked akinesia without rigidity. The reaction time paradigm has later been used extensively in clinical-neurophysiological studies in parkinsonian patients, but with inhomogenous results. Given the large variability in the expression of symptoms, and medication problems, this is not surprising. But, on the whole, it emerged that reaction times are more often normal than not, which seems odd in view of the frequent sign of bradykinesia. The clue lies in the clinical observation that it is movement self-initiation which is disturbed in parkinsonian patient rather than sensory-triggered movements. Studies in parkinsonian patients contributed a lot to the notion that self-initiatiated and sensory triggered or guided movements depend on different mechanisms and neural structures. With the reaction time paradigm, it is possible to manipulate and to challenge preparatory or cognitive aspects of a movement task by using specific instructions during a delay (waiting) period. The predictive value can then be measured in the result of the forthcoming response.

Readiness to Move
With EEG methods, gross potential changes can be recorded over wide areas of the cerebral cortex during the waiting period, the so-called contingent negative variations or

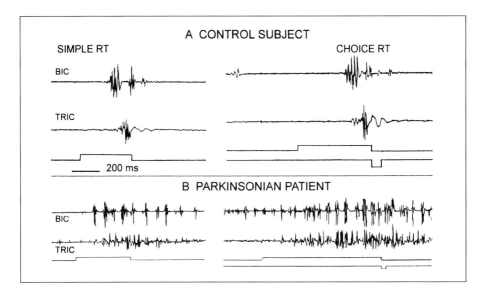

Fig. 10. EMG and mechanic assessment of reaction time (RT) in a control subject and a parkinsonian patient (from Wiesendanger et al. [47]). On the left simple RT, on the right choice RT. Recordings are from the antagonistic biceps and triceps muscles. Signal below indicates occurrence of visual 'go' signal (upward deflection) and of goal-reaching (downward deflection). The lowest signal in choice RT indicates correct response. Note clear-cut 3-phasic burst pattern in the normal subject and the prolonged, rhythmic activity in the parkinsonian patient without reciprocal 3-phasic bursts.

expectancy waves. In this context, one should mention Richard Jung (1911–1986) who was deeply impressed by the demonstration of Hess that movements and posture are mentally prepared. It was in Jung's laboratory, under his guidance and personal involvement, that the 'Bereitschaftspotentiale' (readiness potentials), occurring before onset of self-initiated movements [116], and the 'Zielpotentiale' (goal-related potentials) were discovered [117]. Jung had an unusal integrative view of motor control and, without training in psychology, had also an exceptionally good knowledge of the older concepts of mental processes of set and readiness which precede movement execution [118]. This is well illustrated in polygraphic recordings of punching or pointing movements (fig. 11) which included the cortical correlates of readiness and goal achievement, the visual 'grasp' of the object, representative EMG activity of muscles related to transport and final phase of the arm movement, EMG activity of anticipatory postural adjustments, and the platform output, signalling stance regulation [119, 120].

Kinematography and the Principle of Motor Equivalence
A radical departure from the traditional study in anesthetized and reduced animal preparations began with the introduction of photographic movement analysis towards the end of the last century. This occurred almost at the same time by Eadweard Muybridge (1830–1904) in the United States and by the physiologist Etienne-Jules Marey (1830–1904) in Paris. This work surely was motivated by the sheer pleasure of looking in detail as complex behavioral acts unfold. But it was also the first scientific approach to kinesiology. The wonderful pictures of the untrained girl throwing a ball contrasting with the expert

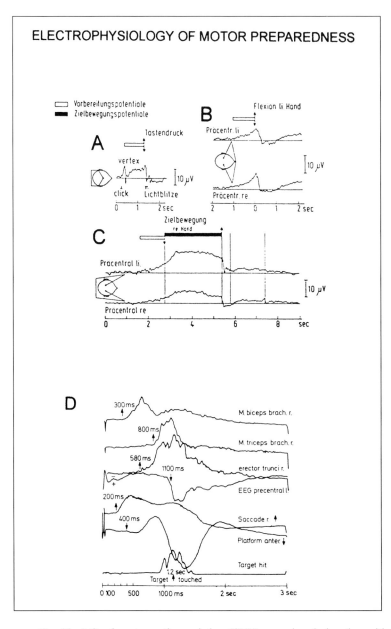

Fig. 11. A Contingent negative variation (CNV) occurring during the waiting period which starts with a click and ends with the visual 'go' signal. **B** Readiness potential starting about 1.5 s before onset of a self-initiated movement. **C** Goal potential ('Zielpotential'), preceded by readiness potential, occurring during the performance of a goal-directed hand movement. **D** EMG activation pattern in goal-directed arm movement. Note the early activation of biceps and trunk muscles, starting before the main mover (triceps), as well as the eye movements for goal fixation. Early changes in weight distribution on the stance platform are also seen. The EEG starts with a CNV potential which continues into a goal potential. From Jung [120].

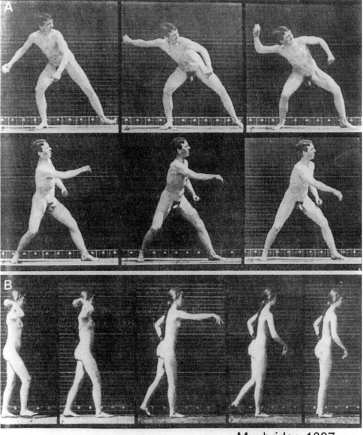

Muybridge 1887

Fig. 12. Movement sequences from a trained sportsman throwing a ball, and from an untrained woman. The comparison shows nicely the involvement of the whole body mass in the trained person to achieve the maximum momentum for throwing the ball. From Muybridge, reproduced in Jung [120].

posture of the trained person (fig. 12) need no further comments. By adding white stripes on black clothes, Marey inaugurated the first stick diagrams which show nicely the cooperative actions of the various body parts, including the postural accompaniments (fig. 13). These studies were an important step forward towards modern research in motor control.

The theoretical dividends of such an approach to motor control came out of the work of Nikolai Alexandrowitch Bernstein (1896–1966). As a young, scientifically-minded physician, Bernstein was appointed in 1922 by the Soviet government to head a new laboratory of biomechanics in order to investigate how the efficiency of manual labor can be increased and optimized (fig. 14). This was the starting point for collecting a large amount of data on how human subjects perform manual professional skills. Most of these include rhythmic arm movements, like striking with a hammer. For analyzing the mechanics, he developed a technique for recording the repetitively performed trajectories, what he

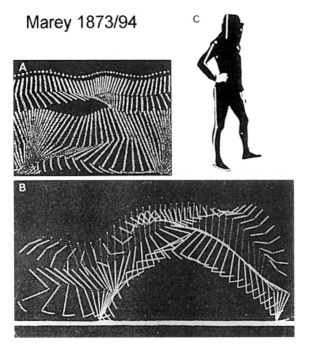

Marey 1873/94

Fig. 13. First stick diagrams of movement sequences obtained by Marey (from Jung [120]). **A** Normal gait. **B** Jumping over an obstacle. Note the coordinated action of the whole body. **C** Momentary positions of head, trunk and limbs are provided by the painted white lines on the black suit (the head line is omitted in **A** and **B**).

called the 'cyclograms'. One generalization he made was the 'principle of equal simplicity'. He illustrated this with circles performed with the outstretched arm, either in front or sidewards of the subject (fig. 15). In both situations, the circles were performed about the same way, and with the same ease, although the implicated muscles and joints were very different. We do not need to consciously change the selection of actuators, it is all automatic and we are only aware of the goal. Bernstein furthermore observed that goal achievement is relatively invariant compared to the large variability of the individual trajectories. He also illustrates this with superimposed cyclograms, published in the English translation of some of his work [121]. As another example for the principle of equal simplicity, he mentions writing with hand movements, whole arm movements, or with mouth movements. As in the above example, the same goal can be achieved with quite different muscles and joints.

Interestingly, the same example was used by Karl Spencer Lashley (1890–1958) at about the same time [122] for explaining his principle of motor equivalence: two names, the same idea! I do not know whether Lashley and Bernstein knew of each other having described the same principle. But in his 1935 paper 'The Problem of the Interrelation of Co-ordination and Localization' (also reproduced in the 1967 English monograph), Bernstein in fact mentions Lashley's book Brain Mechanisms and Intelligence [123], but only in the context of Lashley's concept of equipotentiality (which Bernstein found erroneous). In any case, the term of *motor equivalence* is now well established in the field of motor control,

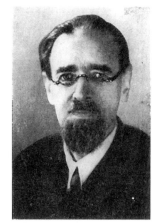

Nikolai Alexandrowitsch Bernstein (1896 - 1966)
Original publication of "THE PROBLEM OF THE
INTERRELATION OF CO-ORDINATION AND LOCALIZATION"
(PROBLEMA VZAIMOOTNOŠENIJ KOORDINACII I LOKALZACII)

ARCHIVES DES SCIENCES BIOLOGIQUES
FONDÉES EN 1892 PAR L'INSTITUT DE MÉDECINE EXPÉRIMENTALE

АРХИВ
БИОЛОГИЧЕСКИХ
НАУК

ОСНОВАН В 1892 г. ИНСТИТУТОМ
ЭКСПЕРИМЕНТАЛЬНОЙ МЕДИЦИНЫ
ИЗДАТЕЛЬСТВО
ВСЕСОЮЗНОГО ИНСТИТУТА ЭКСПЕРИМЕНТАЛЬНОЙ МЕДИЦИНЫ
МОСКВА—1935—ЛЕНИНГРАД

Fig. 14. Portrait of Nikolai Alexandrowitsch Bernstein (reproduced from Bernstein, 1987) and first page of the important original paper of Bernstein on coordination and localization, published in 1935 (later translated in English and published as chapter 2 in Bernstein [121]). The reprint was dedicated by Bernstein to Dr. Mark Shik (who gave it to the author in 1991).

particularly since goal-oriented movements, such as reaching and grasping an object, are now so intensely studied [e.g. 124]. It can be defined as invariant goal achievement with variable means [125]. It is also worth mentioning that Lashley (122) derived the motor equivalence principle primarily from observations on rats and monkeys subjected to brain lesions and whose score were not different from control animals. It is important to realize that Lashley was interested in the score of task performance, in essence the number of errors made by the animals. The learned tasks consisted in finding the path in a maze for the rats and in manipulative skills for monkeys; the detailed parameters of movement components were, however, not taken into account. In other words, Lashley was interested in assessing the higher-order control of goal achievement, not the lower level deficits of movement parameters. Thus the message regarding the outcome of his lesion experiments is that the animal rapidly learned to use still functioning effectors to achieve the goal, but it does not mean that the animals had no deficits (in fact the monkeys did show paretic deficits).

Here one can again learn a lesson which bears on the ongoing controversies about lesion effects of a given structure, such as the motor cortical-pyramidal system. When assessing the score of goal achievement, one may conclude that recovery is rapid and complete. If on the contrary the observer is searching for parametric changes in the exact use of the body parts, he may well find, and over a prolonged time, a number of deficits, such as slowing of movements.

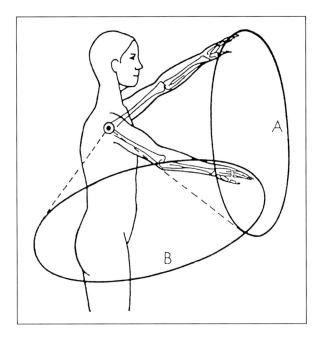

Fig. 15. The outstretched arm performs with the same ease and perfection circles in front of the body and more laterally. This example is given by Bernstein in the paper published in 1935 (see figure 23) to illustrate the *'principle of equal simplicity'* which corresponds to Lashley's *'principle of motor equivalence'*. It says that the same movement project (goal) can be performed with very different means, i.e. innervation patterns.

The notion of motor equivalence is in my opinion a crucial concept, not only in motor control research, but also in practical neurological rehabilitation: therapists indeed pay particular attention to still functioning actuators that may be trained to perform an equivalent job for a given goal. Lashley also emphasized the importance of motivation as a factor influencing the performance score. He found that, compared to controls, motivation in lesioned animals is less stable, with large day-by-day variability. Self-observations of neuroscientists recovering from hemiparesis after stroke are moving descriptions of the enormous mental strain to initiate a voluntary movement of the paretic limb, as well as of the increased fatiguability [126, 127].

The study of higher motor control obviously invites a top-down approach. But there is no need to oppose top-down and bottom-up strategies, both having their advantages and limitations. As long as there are still so many gaps in our knowledge, it is probably wise to work on both levels. Paul Weiss [128], a developmental biologist, made this point very clear in his discussion on the stratified nature of biological systems. His definition of a system is that it has a smaller variance (V_{syst}) than the sum of the variances (V) of its constituents a, b, c, ...n; i.e:

$$V_{syst} < S\{V_a, V_b, V_c ... V_n\}.$$

This means '... *that the elements ... are subject to restraints of their degrees of freedom so as to yield a resultant in the direction of maintaining the optimum stability of the collective.*

The term "coordination", "control", and the like, are synonymous labels for this principle' (p. 12).

This statement of a cellular biologist comes astonishingly near to the motor equivalence principle of Lashley; it conforms with the notion of invariant goal achievement with variable means. One might ask whether such a principle is not too general for being of any heuristic value. I don't believe so. It would be very difficult, practically impossible, to assess coordination of a complex multiarticulate synergy in terms of all possible movement parameters and muscle actions.

In a behavioral study in monkeys, conditioned to perform a bimanual pull-and-grasp task, we have shown that it is possible to assess quantitatively, and with relatively simple time measurements, the score in goal coordination [129]. The remarkable dichotomy in control levels was demonstrated by changing task constraints: when vision was excluded, we observed a highly significant slowing in the two hand movements (fig. 16A). However, synchronization of the two hands was perfectly maintained, and the paired times of goal-reaching remained highly correlated (fig. 16B). Therefore, we concluded that the changed timing parameters, the variable means, still covaried, resulting in the observed invariant goal achievement. We have also observed dramatic changes in the timing structure of the same task as a result of cortical lesions with preserved goal achievement (to be reported separately). This is similar to what Lashley [130] described in his monkeys with precentral lesions: recovery with immediate adaptive changes in the use of the limbs for opening the boxes, and given the problems occurring with antiparkinsonian medication, allowing them to recover their preoperative score; in other words, preserved goal achievement with changed (paretic) movements.

The top-down approach relies on the concept of a 'downward causation' implying that there is a gradually developing control that constrains the lower components progressively together as the moving limbs (or limb segments) approach the goal. In our experimental situation, evidence for such a coordinative structure was expressed in a relatively invariant synchronization with high correlation coefficients in the arrival times of the two limbs. We still ignore the mechanisms that would explain preservation of goal achievement. Our present working hypothesis is that feed-forward proprioceptive signals of the leading arm are generated which then are used by internal (cortical) representations to update the course of the other hand.

Conclusion

After having gone through some of the older literature concerning human motor control, with an attempt to follow the development from the early concepts to the present era of research in this field, the question naturally arises: What were the ideas which most influenced the field of human motor control? I have enumerated some of the technical reasons which partly explain the increasing pace of progress in this field. Perhaps as important, however, was the move to nonreduced preparations and, not least, the choice to study goal-oriented movements in human subjects. It led to the insight that mental accompaniments of goal identification, planning a strategy, decision-making, attention, motivation, readiness, motor memory and anticipation of the motion's effect, in short all so-called cognitive aspects, are integrated components of motor control. This pertains of course also to motor control in animals, especially in subhuman primates, but it is in humans that these functions reached their highest development and that these factors may be manipulated without long-lasting training procedures. For motor neuroscientists, the

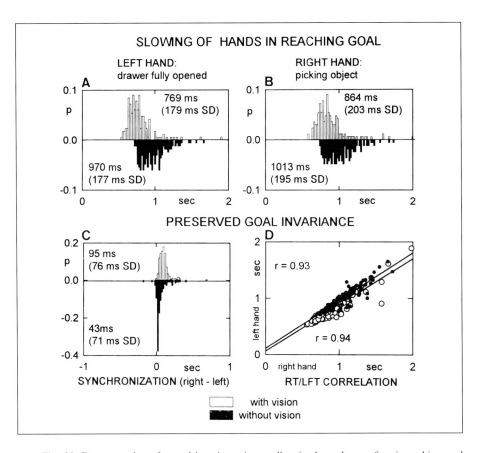

Fig. 16. Demonstration of a goal invariance in a well-trained monkey performing a bimanual pull-and-grasp synergy, either with vision (upward histograms) or without vision (downward histograms). **A** and **B** are time histograms of arrival time of, respectively, the left and the right hands at the goal. **C** shows histograms of paired intervals (**A–B**) as a measure of synchronization. **D** are regression plots of paired left hand and right hand arrival times with correlation coefficients. Note the pronounced slowing when the monkey performed in the dark. This contrasts with the maintained goal invariance, expressed in the good synchronization and in the high correlation coefficient. From experiments of Kazennikov et al. [129].

book of Evarts et al. [109] on 'Neurophysiological Approaches to Higher Brain Functions' was a milestone and an eye-opener. Only very few neurophysiologists had so far dared to approach these higher spheres of motor control. Through his early association with Lashley, Ed Evarts knew about psychological concepts which neurophysiologists were hardly familiar with, or tended to ignore. One central issue which guided Evarts work for the last 10 years of his life was the search for neuronal correlates of set. Many followed him since. Evarts also recognized that some problems of 'motor psychophysics' can more easily be tested in human subjects and neurological patients, and that is also what he did. The timely intrusion of psychological concepts in the field of motor control since the early 70s is a recent story; the impact of Evarts and many others which since continue to explore this fascinating field is overwhelming.

As usual, however, a new direction in research does not come out of nothing. As I tried to demonstrate, there were a few forerunners who strongly advocated the need of bringing together concepts of physiology and psychology in motor control and of studying motor control in animals which are free to move and also in human subjects, rather than in reduced and anesthetized preparations. The work of Hoffmann and of Wachholder (who were rather isolated in the then current field of neurophysiology) went unnoticed outside Germany, and it was only 30 and 50 years later that this pioneeering work was rediscovered and appreciated. Hoffmann's work was rediscovered outside Germany; Wachholder's and Altenburger's involvement in motor control was perhaps too short to produce any major impact. Today, they are at least cited for their description of the reciprocal 3-burst pattern of antagonistic muscle pairs in fast voluntary movements (which represents only a small fraction of the conceptual richness of their work). The pioneering EMG studies of Altenburger and Foerster on the pathophysiology of intentional movements left almost no traces. It is only in recent years, i.e. 70 years later, that this research domain florishes again. The legacy of the Vogts is their far-sighted multidisciplinary approach to brain research. They will be remembered for their first combined structural-functional parcellation of the cerebral cortex which led to the notion of primary, secondary and even tertiary motor fields. In spite of the critique of an exaggerated parcellation, this work had a major impact through its practical application in neurosurgery by Foerster and, through him, by Penfield and Jasper. Jung's legacy as a neurologist is his life-long endeavor to apply electrophysiological techniques for objective assessment of neurological disorders of oculomotricity, posture, tremor and sleep, as well as his keen interest and support in studies of movement preparation.

These neuroscientists have something in common: their research approach was not conventional, the reception by colleagues often skeptical, but from today's perspective of course innovative. Why did it take so long for this work to really begin to influence and to change the emphasis in motor control research? There may be several reasons, but one is very likely the disastrous political developments in Germany which began soon after much of the described research had been done, and then the war. At the end of the war, Hoffmann who was already somewhat isolated in his research, was without any collaborator, three of them being killed in the war, the institute bombed out. The Vogts were forced to leave their Brain Research Institute and lived in reduced facilities and in the isolation of the Black Forest. Wachholder gave up his research in motor control as he moved to Rostock in 1933 where he seemed to have been more and more absorbed by administrative charges and by the troubles of regime and then the war. Altenburger died very young. Through his many excellent handbook articles and international contacts, Foerster was the most charismatic of all. But with the Nazi regime began also a difficult time for him; several of his collaborators had to leave the Foerster institute because they were Jewish and he and his wife, also of Jewish origin, were in danger. The last years until his death in 1941, he lived also in relative isolation. Bernstein was politically isolated from the Western world where he was only discovered after the translation and publication of his book on the Co-ordination and Regulation of Movements [121], and later through publications of his associate Viktor S. Gurfinkel and his school who carried on with research in human motor control in the spirit of Bernstein.

Last but not least, my admiration goes to Walter Rudolph Hess for his contributions which are marked by great originality. Although, as a Swiss citizen, he escaped the atrocities of the war, communications with colleagues in Europe were much reduced during this time. In spite of a modest financial budget and with only a few collaborators, he remained a very productive researcher, and this besides his heavy teaching duties. His integrative

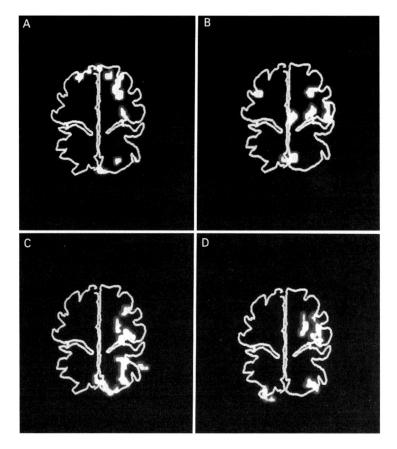

Fig. 17. Noninvasive brain imaging (PET scans) illustrating the widely distributed activation pattern of sensorimotor areas produced by subjects performing a complex motor task. Shown are the averaged differences (rest–task), obtained in 10 healthy subjects. In this experiment, subjects were requested to point in a defined sequence to 7 targets distributed in the peripersonal space. The targets were circles of varying diameters. These targets were visible only for a brief period and subjects had to point from memory to the targets after a variable delay of about 90 s ('delayed reaching task'). Thus the paradigm consists of a preparatory delay phase and an execution phase. Since the sequence has to be repeated many times, one can furthermore postulate a learning process. The 4 maps represent activation patterns obtained during the delay period in **A** and **B**, and during the execution phase in **C** and **D**. At the beginning of the learning process, images **A** and **C** were obtained, when the sequence was well learned, the images **B** and **D**. Three remarkable conclusions can be made: (1) the purely mental process of movement preparation results already in multiple activated foci, including also the motor cortex; (2) transition from preparation to action results in a marked dynamic change in the activation pattern (comparison **A**+**B** with **C**+**D**), and (3) there is also a remarkable redistribution in the transition from the learning phase to well-practiced motor behavior (comparison **A**+**C** with **B**+**D**). Experiments performed by Kawashima, et al. [J Neurosci 1994;14, reproduced with permission].

view on motor control has many common features with that of Bernstein, and in some respect also of Lashley. Although Hess was rewarded with the Nobel prize in 1949, his truly innovative research approach has been somewhat forgotten, even so his ideas sound remarkably modern (see below). Part of his writings are now available through a recent translation and publication of a book edited by his pupil Konrad Akert [26].

I think there is no better way to close this chapter than by reproducing summarizing views on motricity as written by Hess in his last book 'A Biological View of Psychology' [131]. He concludes the chapter on intentional movements with the following 5 points (my nonverbatim and slightly shortened translation): (1) An intentional action is induced by a conscious drive and set. (2) The perception of the object in a goal-oriented movement and its memorized content contribute to the drive and motivation for prehension. (3) A manyfold of innervation pattern characterizes the probing of the limb. (4) Goal achievement reinforces the used innervation pattern, thus steadily improving the performance by learning. (5) Disturbances of central coordination are compensated adaptatively.

His final conclusion is that the organization of a goal-oriented actions is not implemented within one localized center, but it requires widely distributed and interrelated neural networks of cortical as well as subcortical structures which all have to cooperate in fulfilling the goal of the action plan. Today, we can indeed visualize this distributed activation pattern in PET scans which correspond amazingly well with the inferences of Hess (fig. 17).

References

1   Hoffmann P: Die physiologischen Eigenschaften der Eigenreflexe. Ergeb Physiol 1934;36:15–108.
2   Piper: Die Aktionsströme menschlicher Muskeln. Z Biol Tech Methoden 1913;3:52.
3   Hoffmann P: Beiträge zur Kenntnis der menschlichen Reflexe mit besonderer Berücksichtigung der elektrischen Erscheinungen. Arch Anat Physiol 1910:223–246.
4   Creed RS, Denny-Brown D, Eccles JC, Liddell EGT: Reflex Activity of the Spinal Cord. Oxford, Clarendon Press, 1932, pp 1–184.
5   Liddell EGT: The Discovery of Reflexes. Oxford, Clarendon Press, 1960.
6   Jung R: Paul Hoffmann 1884–1962. Ergeb Physiol 1969;61:1–17.
7   Lloyd DPC: Conduction and synaptic transmission of the reflex response to stretch in spinal cats. J Neurophysiol 1943;6:317–326.
8   Magladery JW, McDougal DB: Electrophysiological studies of nerve and reflex activity in normal man. I. Identification of certain reflexes in the electromyogram and the conduction velocity of peripheral nerve fibers. Johns Hopkins Hosp Bull 1950;86:265–290.
9   Paillard J: Analyse électrophysiologique et comparaison, chez l'Homme, du réflexe de Hoffmann et du réflexe myotatique. Pflügers Arch Ges Physiol 1955;260:448–479.
10 Magladery JW: Some observations on spinal reflexes in man. Pflügers Arch Ges Physiol 1955;261:302–321.
11 Tanaka R: Reciprocal Ia inhibition during voluntary movements in man. Exp Brain Res 1974;21: 529–540.
12 Pierrot-Deseilligny E, Mazières L: Spinal mechanisms underlying spasticity; in Delwaide PJ, Young RR (eds): Clinical Neurophysiology in Spasticity. Amsterdam, Elsevier, 1985, pp 63–76.
13 Delwaide PJ, Young RR: Clinical Neurophysiology in Spasticity. Amsterdam, Elsevier, 1985.
14 Hultborn H, Meunier S, Morin C, Pierrot-Deseilligny E: Assessing changes in presynaptic inhibition of Ia fibres: A study in man and the cat. J Physiol (Lond) 1987;389:729–756.
15 Bussel B, Pierrot-Deseilligny E: Inhibition of human motoneurones, probably of Renshaw origin, elicited by an orthodromic motor discharge. J Physiol (Lond) 1977;269:319–339.
16 Gurfinkel V, Kots JM, Shik ML: The regulation of human posture (in Russian). Moscow, Nauka, 1965.
17 Kots YM: The Organization of Voluntary Movement: Neurophysiological Mechanisms. New York, Plenum, 1977.
18 Gurfinkel VS, Kots JM, Paltsev FI, Feldman AG: Models of the Structural Functional Organization of Certain Biological Systems. Cambridge/Mass, MIT Press, 1971, pp 382–395.
19 Eichenberger A, Rüegg DG: Relation between the specific H-reflex facilitation preceding a voluntary movement and movement parameters in man. J Physiol 1984;347:545–559.
20 Katz R, Meunier S, Pierrot-Deseilligny E: Changes in presynaptic inhibition of Ia fibres in man while standing. Brain 1988;111:417–437.
21 Stein RB, Capaday C: The modulation of human reflexes during functional motor tasks. Trends Neurosci 1988; 11:328–332.
22 Liddell EGT, Sherrington CS: Reflexes in response to stretch (myotatic reflexes). Proc R Soc Lond [B] 1924; 96:212–242.
23 Magnus R: Körperstellung. Berlin, Springer, 1924.
24 Rademaker GGJ: Experimentelle Physiologie des Hirnstammes (mit Ausnahme der vegetativen Funktionen); in Bumke O, Foerster O (eds): Handbuch der Neurologie: Allgemeine Neurologie. II. Experimentelle Physiologie. Berlin, Springer, 1927, pp 187–234.

25   Gahéry Y: Associated movements, postural adjustments and synergies: Some comments about the history and significance of three motor concepts. Arch Ital Biol 1987;125:345–360.

26   Akert K: Biological Order and Brain Organization; Selected Works of W.R. Hess. Berlin, Springer, 1981, pp 1–347.

27   Jung R: Walter R. Hess (1881–1973). Rev Physiol Biochem Pharmacol 1981;88:1–21.

28   Jung R, Hassler R: The extrapyramidal motor system; in Field J, Magoun HW, Hall VE (eds): Handbook of Physiology, sect 1: Neurophysiology, vol II. Washington, Americal Physiological Society, 1960, pp 863–927.

29   Belenki VY, Gurfinkel VS, Paltsev YI: Elements of control of voluntary movements. Biofizika 1967;12: 135–141.

30   Nashner LM, McCollum G: The organization of human postural movements: A formal basis and experimental synthesis. Behav Brain Sci 1985;8:135–172.

31   Massion J: Movement, posture and equilibrium: Interaction and coordination. Prog Neurobiol 1992;38:35–56.

32   Granit R: Some comments on 'tone'; in Granit R, Pompeiano O (eds): Reflex Control of Movements. Prog Brain Res. Amsterdam, Elsevier, 1979, vol 50, pp XVII–XIX (opening lecture).

33   Mori S, Kawahara K, Sakamoto T, Aoki M, Tomiyama T: Setting and resetting of level of postural muscle tone in decerebrate cat by stimulation of brain stem. J Neurophysiol 1982;48:737–748.

34   Hounsgaard J, Hultborn H, Kiehn O: Transmitter-controlled properties of alpha-motoneurones causing long-lasting motor discharge to brief excitatory inputs. Prog Brain Res 1986;64:39–49.

35   Wiesendanger M, Palmeri A, Corboz M: Some pathophysiological considerations about muscle tone and spasticity; in Benecke R, Davidoff RA, Emre M (eds): The Origin and Treatment of Spasticity. Carnforth, Parthenon, 1990, pp 15–27.

36   Wiesendanger M, Hummelsheim H, Bianchetti M, Chen DF, Hyland B, Maier V, Wiesendanger R: Input and output organization of the supplementary motor area; in Bock G, O'Connor M, Marsh J (eds): Motor Areas of the Cerebral Cortex. Ciba Symp No 132. Chichester, Wiley, 1987, pp 40–62.

37   Chen DF, Hyland B, Maier V, Palmeri A, Wiesendanger M: Comparison of neural activity in the supplementary motor cortex and in the primary motor cortex in monkeys performing a choice-reaction task. Somatosens Mot Res 1991;8:27–44.

38   Mellah S, Rispal-Padel L, Riviere G: Changes in excitability of motor units during preparation for movement. Exp Brain Res 1990;82:178–186.

39   Wachholder K: Willkürliche Haltung und Bewegung. Ergeb Physiol 1928;26:568–775.

40   Kohnstamm O: Über Koordination, Tonus und Hemmung. Z Diät Phys Ther 1901;4:112–122.

41   Foerster O: Die Physiologie und Pathologie der Koordination. Monatsschr Psychiatr 1902;5.

42   Fessard A: Le Mouvement Volontaire, d'après K. Wachholder. Paris, Chahine, 1926, pp 1–69.

43   Fessard A: Allocution inaugurale. Int Symp Motor Aspects of Behaviour and Programmed Nervous Activities. Brain Res 1974;71:V–XI.

44   Tournay A, Fessard A: Analyse électromyographique de quelques mouvements volontaires. Ass Fr Avanc Sci 1948;145:514–517.

45   Livingston RB, Paillard J, Tournay A, Fessard A: Plasticité d'une synergie musculaire dans l'exécution d'un mouvement volontaire. J Physiol (Paris) 1951;43:605–619.

46   Paillard J: The patterning of skilled movements; in Field J, Magoun HW, Hall VE (eds): Handbook of Physiology, sect 1: Neurophysiology, vol II. Washington, American Physiological Society, 1960, pp 1679–1708.

47   Wiesendanger M, Schneider P, Villoz JP: Elektromyographische Analyse der raschen Willkürbewegung. Schweiz Arch Neurol Neurochir Psychiatr 1967;100:88–99.

48   Angel RW: Electromyography during voluntary movement: The two-burst pattern. Electroencephalogr Clin Neurophysiol 1974;36:493–498.

49   Ghez C, Gordon J: Trajectory control in targeted force impulses. I. Role of opposing muscles. Exp Brain Res 1987;67:225–240.

50   Meinck HM, Benecke R, Meyer W, Höhne J, Conrad B: Human ballistic finger flexion: Uncoupling of the three-burst pattern. Exp Brain Res 1984;55:127–133.

51   Sanes JN, Jennings VA: Centrally programmed patterns of muscle activity in voluntary motor behavior of humans. Exp Brain Res 1984;54:23–32.

52   Brown SHC, Cooke JD: Amplitude- and instruction-dependent modulation of movement-related electromyogram activity in humans. J Physiol (Lond) 1981;316:97–107.

53   Lestienne F: Effects of inertial load and velocity on the breaking process of voluntary limb movements. Exp Brain Res 1979;35:407–418.

54   Hallett M, Shahani BT, Young RR: EMG analysis of stereotyped voluntary movements in man. J Neurol Neurosurg Psychiatry 1975;38:1154–1162.

55   Gordon J, Ghez C: Trajectory control in targeted force impulses. II. Pulse height control. Exp Brain Res 1987; 67:241–252.

56   Hufschmidt JH, Hufschmidt T: Antagonist inhibition as the earliest sign of a sensory-motor reaction. Nature 1954;174:607.

57   Conrad B, Benecke R, Goehmann M: Premovement silent period in fast movement initiation. Exp Brain Res 1983;51:310–313.

58   Yabe K: Premotion silent period in rapid voluntary movement. J Appl Physiol 1976;41:470–473.

59   Evarts EV: Activity of the motor cortex neurons in association with learned movement. Int J Neurosci 1972; 3:113–124.

60   Jongen HAH, Denier van der Gon JJ, Gielen CCAM: Inhomogeneous activation of motoneurone pools as revealed by co-contraction of antagonistic human arm muscles. Exp Brain Res 1989;75:555–562.

61   Liddell EGT, Sherrington CS: Recruitment and some other features of reflex inhibition. Proc R Soc Lond [B] 1925;97:488–518.

62   Schlapp M: Observations on a voluntary tremor – violinist's vibrato. Q J Exp Physiol 1973;58:357–368.

63   Lippold OCJ: Oscillation in the stretch reflex arc and the origin of the rhythmical, 8–12 c/s component of physiological tremor. J Physiol 1970;206:359–382.

64   Matthews PBC, Muir RB: Comparison of electromyogram spectra with force spectra during human elbow tremor. J Physiol 1980;302:427–441.

65   Burne JA, Lippold OCJ, Pryor M: Proprioceptors and normal tremor. J Physiol 1984;348:559–572.

66   Brown TIH, Rack PMH, Ross HF: Different types of tremor in the human thumb. J Physiol 1982;332:113–123.

67   Elble R, Randall JE: Motor unit activity responsible for 8–12 Hz component of human physiological tremor. J Neurophysiol 1976;39:370–383.

68   Hagbarth KE, Young RR: Participation of the stretch reflex in human physiological tremor. Brain 1979;102: 509–526.

69   Vallbo AB, Wessberg JP: Organization of motor output in slow finger movements in man. J Physiol (Lond) 1993;469:673–691.

70   Wessberg JP, Vallbo AB, Lang E: Coding of pulsatile motor output by human muscle afferents during slow finger movements. J Physiol (Lond) 1995;485:271–282.

71   Welsh JP, Lang EJ, Sugihara I, Llinas R: Dynamic organization of motor control within the olivocerebellar system. Nature 1995;374:453–457.

72   Kelso JAS: Dynamic Patterns – The Self-Organization of Brain and Behavior. Cambridge/Mass, MIT Press, 1985, pp 1–334.

73   De Montigny C, Lamarre Y: Rhythmic activity induced by harmaline in the olivocerebellar-bulbar system of the cat. Brain Res 1973;53:81–95.

74   Kornmüller AE: Über einige bei Willkürbewegungen und auf Sinnesreize auftretende bioelektrische Erscheinungen der Hirnrinde des Menschen. Z Sinnesphysiol 1940;68:121–149.

75   Jasper H, Penfield W: Electrocorticogram in man: Effect of the voluntary movement upon the electrical activity of the precentral gyrus. Arch Psychiatr Z Neurol 1949;183:163–174.

76   Pfurtscheller G: Central beta-rhythm during sensorimotor activity in man. Electroencephalogr Clin Neurophysiol 1981;51:253–264.

77   Pfurtscheller G, Berghold A: Patterns of cortical activation during planning of voluntary movement. Electroencephalogr Clin Neurophysiol 1989;72:250–258.

78   Pfurtscheller G, Neuper C, Kalcher J: 40-Hz oscillations during motor behavior in man. Neurosci Lett 1993; 164:179–182.

79   Kristeva-Feige R, Feige B, Makeig S, Ross B, Elbert T: Oscillatory brain activity during a motor task. Neuroreport 1993;4:1291–1294.

80   Chen DF: Synaptic interactions between primate cortical neurons revealed by in vitro intracellular potentials; PhD thesis, Univ Washington, Seattle 1993, pp 1–159.

81   Sanes JN, Donoghue JP: Oscillations in local field potentials of the primate motor cortex during voluntary movement. Proc Natl Acad Sci USA 1993;90:4470–4474.

82   Murthy VN, Fetz EE: Coherent 25- to 35-Hz oscillations in the sensorimotor cortex of awake behaving monkeys. Proc Natl Acad Sci USA 1992;89:5670–5674.

83   Nashmi R, Mendonça K, MacKay WA: EEG rhythms of the sensorimotor region during hand movements. Electroencephalogr Clin Neurophysiol 1994;91:456–467.

84   Toro C, Cox C, Friehs G, Ojakangas C, Maxwell R, Gates JR, Gumnit RJ, Ebner TJ: 8–12 Hz rhythmic oscillations in human motor cortex during two-dimensional arm movements: Evidence for representation of kinematic parameters. Electroencephalogr Clin Neurophysiol Electromyogr Motor Control 1994;93:390–403.

85   Zülch KJ: Otfried Foerster; in Kolle K (ed): Grosse Nervenärzte. Stuttgart, Thieme, 1970, vol 1, pp 81–98.

86   Sherrington C: The Integrative Action of the Nervous System, ed 2. New Haven, Yale University Press, 1947, pp 1–413.

87   Foerster O: On the indication and results of the excision of posterior spinal nerve roots in man. Surg Gynecol Obstet 1913;16:463–474.

88   Sindou M, Jeanmonod D, Mertens P: Surgery in the dorsal root entry-zone: Microsurgical DREZ-tomy (MDT) for the treatment of spasticity; in Sindou M, Abbott R, Keravel Y (eds): Neurosurgery for Spasticity – A Multidisciplinary Approach. Wien, Springer, 1981, pp 165–182.

89   Foerster O: Motorische Felder und Bahnen; in Bumke O, Foerster O (eds): Handbuch der Neurologie. VI. Berlin, Springer, 1936a, pp 1–357.

90   Foerster O: The motor cortex in man in the light of Hughlings Jackson's doctrines. Brain 1936;59:135–159.

91   Kennard MA: Somatic functions; in Bucy PC (ed): The Precentral Motor Cortex. Urbana, The University of Illinois Press, 1944, pp 243–276.

92   Altenburger H: Elektrodiagnostik (einschliesslich Chronaxie und Aktionsströmen); in Bumke O, Foerster O (eds): Handbuch der Neurologie. Berlin, Springer, 1937, pp 747–1096.

93   Walshe FMR: La rigidité décérébrée de Sherrington et ses relations avec la rigidité musculaire d'origine pyramidale chez l'homme. Encephale 1925;20:73–88.

94   Evarts EV: Sherrington's concept of proprioception. Trends Neurosci 1981;Feb:44–46.

95   Kreutzberg GW, Klatzo I, Kleihues P: Oskar and Cècile Vogt, Lenin's brain and the bumble-bees of the Black Forest: Historical note. Brain Pathol 1992;2:363–371.

96   Jung R: Some European neuroscientists: A personal tribute; in Worden FG, Swazey JP, Adelman G (eds): The Neurosciences: Paths of Discovery. Cambridge/Mass, MIT Press, 1993, pp 477–517.

97   Hassler R: Cécile und Oskar Vogt; in Kolle K (ed): Grosse Nervenärzte, Stuttgart, Thieme, 1970, vol 2, pp 45–64.

98   Vogt C, Vogt O: Die vergleichend-architektonische und die vergleichend-reizphysiologische Felderung der Grosshirnrinde unter besonderer Berücksichtigung der menschlichen. Naturwissenschaften 1926;14:1190–1194.

99   Foerster O, Penfield W: The structural basis of traumatic epilepsy and results of radical operation. Brain 1930; 53:99–119.

100   Penfield W, Jasper H: Epilepsy and the Functional Anatomy of the Human Brain. Boston; Little, Brown, 1954.

101   Talairach J, Bancaud J: The supplementary motor area in man (anatomo-functional findings by stereoencephalography in epilepsy). Int J Neurol 1966;5:330–347.

102   Wiesendanger M: Recent developments in studies of the supplementary motor area of primates. Rev Physiol Biochem Pharmacol 1986;103:1–59.

103   Wiesendanger M: The riddle of supplementary motor area function; in Mano N, Hamada I, DeLong MR (eds): Role of the Cerebellum and Basal Ganglia in Voluntary Movement. Amsterdam, Elsevier, 1993, pp 253–266.

104   Lüders HO: The supplementary sensorimotor area. New York, Raven Press, 1995, pp 1–575.

105   Donders FC: Die Schnelligkeit psychischer Prozesse. Arch Anat Physiol 1968:657–666.

106   Exner S: Experimentelle Untersuchung der einfachsten psychischen Prozesse. 1. Abhandlung: Die persönliche Gleichung. Pflügers Arch Ges Physiol 1873;7:601–609.

107   Kraepelin E: Memoirs (translated from German). Berlin, Springer, 1987, pp 1–270.

108   Gibson JJ: A critical review of the concept of set in contemporary experimental psychology. Psychol Bull 1941; 38:781–817.

109   Evarts EV, Shinoda Y, Wise SP: Neurophysiological Approaches to Higher Brain Functions. New York, Wiley, 1984, pp 1–198.

110   Prochazka A: Sensorimotor gain control: A basic strategy of motor systems? (Review). Prog Neurobiol 1989; 33:281–307.

111   Vörckel H: Reaktionszeit der willkürlichen Kontraktion und Erschlaffung der Beuger und Strecker des Vorderarmes. Z Biol 1922;75:79.

112   Wirth W: Die Reaktionszeiten; in Bethe A, von Bergmann G, Embden G, Ellinger A (eds): Handbuch der normalen und pathologischen Physiologie: Spezielle Physiologie des Zentralnervensystems der Wirbeltiere. Springer, Berlin, 1927, pp 525–599.

113   Welford AT: Reaction Times. London, Academic Press, 1980, pp 1–417.

114   Meyer DE, Osman AM, Irwin DE, Yantis S: Modern mental chronometry. Biol Psychol 1988;26:3–67.

115   Glickstein M: Brain mechanisms in reaction time. Brain Res 1972;40:33–37.

116   Kornhuber HH, Deecke L: Hirnpotentialänderungen bei Willkürbewegungen und passiven Bewegungen des Menschen: Bereitschaftspotential und reafferente Potentiale. Pflügers Arch Ges Physiol 1965;284:1–17.

117   Grünewald-Zuberbier E, Grünewald G, Jung R: Slow potentials of the human precentral and parietal cortex during goal-directed movements (Zielbewegungspotentiale). J Physiol (Lond) 1978;284:181–182.

118   Creutzfeldt O: Richard Jung (1911–1986). Exp Brain Res 1986;64:1–4.

119   Jung R: Postural support of goal-directed movements: The preparation and guidance of voluntary action in man. Acta Biol Acad Sci Hung 1982;33:201–213.

120   Jung R: Zur Bewegungsphysiologie beim Menschen: Fortbewegung, Zielsteuerung und Sportleistung; in Berger W (ed): Haltung und Bewegung beim Menschen. Berlin, Springer, 1984, pp 7–63.

121   Bernstein NA: The Coordination and Regulation of Movements. Oxford, Pergamon Press, 1967.

122   Lashley KS: Integrative functions of the cerebral cortex. Physiol Rev 1933;13:1–42.

123   Lashley KS: Brain Mechanisms and Intelligence: A Quantitative Study of Injuries to the Brain. Chicago, University of Chicago Press, 1929.

124   Jeannerod M: The neural and behavioural organization of goal-directed movements; in Oxford Psychology Series No 15. Oxford, Clarendon Press, 1988, pp 283–280.

125   Abbs JH, Cole KJ: Neural mechanisms of motor equivalence and goal achievement; in Wise SP (ed): Higher Brain Functions. New York, Wiley, 1987, pp 15–43.

126   Brodal A: Self-observations and neuro-anatomical considerations after a stroke. Brain 1973;96:653–674.

127   Forel A: Subjektive und induktive Selbstbeobachtung über psychische und nervöse Tätigkeit nach Hirnthrombose (oder Apoplexie). J Psychol Neurol 1915;21:145–169.

128   Weiss PA: The living system: Determinism stratified; in Koestler A, Smythies JR (eds): Beyond Reductionism. London, Hutchinson, 1969, pp 3–55.

129   Kazennikov O, Wicki U, Corboz M, Hyland B, Palmeri A, Rouiller EM, Wiesendanger M: Temporal structure of a bimanual goal-directed movement sequence in monkeys. Eur J Neurosci 1994;6:203–210.

130   Lashley KS: Studies in cerebral function in learning. V. The retention of motor habits after destruction of the so-called motor areas in primates. Arch Neurol Psychiatry (Chic) 1924;12:249–276.

131   Hess WR: Psychologie in biologischer Sicht. Stuttgart, Thieme, 1962, pp 1–122.

Dr. Mario Wiesendanger, Neurologische Universitätsklinik,
Motoriklabor BHH-M-130, Inselspital, CH–3010 Bern (Switzerland)

Subject Index

Abduction 94, 95
Acromion markers 48
Action currents 112
Amplitude
  potentials 88
  rhythms 84
Angle changes, movement 47–50
Angular ratios 49, 50
Anodal electric stimulus 91–93
Antagonist activity, muscles 110, 111
Antigravity muscle tone 66, 67
Antisaccadic paradigm 100
Arm raising movement 44
Association areas 10
Atonia, REM sleep 66–70
Auditory evoked potential 80, 81
Automatic movement analysis 53, 54

Balance control during movement 44–50
Basal ganglia 8
Bernstein, Nikolai Alexandrowitch 123–125
Bidimensional movement 10
Bilateral pyramidotomy 5
Bimanual coordination 12, 13
Bodily shifts during sleep 65, 66
Body
  geometry, balance 45
  weight unloading, locomotion training 59, 60,
    62
Brain stimulation 91–101
Bruxism 73
3-Burst pattern, movements 111, 116, 121

Cannabinoids, locomotor activity 62
Center of gravity during movement 44–50
Center of mass during movement 46–49
Central nervous system, center of gravity during
  standing 45–47
Cerebellar nuclei 9

Cerebellum 8
Cerebral cortex, mapping 117, 118
Cerebral imaging 14
Choice reaction time task 81–83
Clonidine, locomotor activity 62, 63
Collaterals 6
Complex movements, analysis 52–56
Contingent negative variation 77–85, 120–122
  spatial distribution 88, 89
Contralateral premotor area 88
Contralateral primary motor area 88
Coordination
  time-based 27, 28
  whole limb 28–30
Cord
  area 2
  dorsum potentials 67, 69
Corpus callosum 98
Cortical excitability during sleep 66
Cortical interneurons during sleep 66
Cortical motor functions 10–12
Corticomotoneuronal fibers 3, 4, 6
Corticospinal axons 6, 33
Corticospinal connectivity 3
Corticospinal neurons 33
Corticospinal projection 96–98
Corticospinal terminations, hand movement 21
Corticospinal tract 8
  rapidly conducting 94, 96
Cranial muscles 96
Cutaneous afferents 12, 27
Cyclograms 124

Degrees of freedom 47, 48
Deltoid muscle 96
Desynchronization 66, 114
Diaphragm 96
Digital dexterity 20
Drugs, locomotor activity 62, 63

EEG
  desynchronization 66, 114
  readiness to move 120–122
  rhythm generation 114
Eigenreflex 104
Electrodes
  epileptic patients 78
  neuronal activity 13, 14
Electromyography 105
  latency 5
  leg muscles 57–64
  posture 108, 110–111
  readiness to move 121, 122
  rhythm generation 112–114, 116
  summation time 5
  walking 54, 55
ELITE system 53, 54
Epileptic patients, cortical potentials 78–89
Epinephrine, locomotor activity 63
Equilibrium control during movement 47–50
ERP 85
Event related desynchronization 84, 87
Eye movement 100

Facial muscles 96, 97
Facilitation-induced latency shortening 93
Fast processor for shape recognition 53, 54
Finger movements
  accuracy 24
  monkeys 3–6
Fingers, independent 20
Flexion-extension 30, 110–113
Fluorescent substances, transport 6
Foerster, Otfried 115–119
Food morsel retrieval test 34–40
Forced grasping 41
Forewarned reaction time task 77
Friction, grip force 25

Gait, analysis 54, 55
Gastrocnemius medialis muscle,
  locomotion 59–63
Goal
  achievement 125
  coordination 127
  invariance 12, 128
Goal-related potentials 121
Go/no-go protocol 81–83
Grasping 12, 27–30
  object attributes 22–27
  visually-directed 19–30
Grip
  formation 22–25
  patterns 19–21
  size 23, 24

timing 28
Grip force 26
  regulation 12
Grip force/load force ratio 25

H-reflex 67, 104, 105
Hamstring activity 54
Hand
  cortical control 21
  grasping 20, 21
  human vs animal 20, 21
  movements 19
    rhythm generation 112–115
  skill 3
Hess, Walter Rudolf 106, 107
Heteronymous monosynaptic reflex 67
Hoffmann, Paul 104, 105
Human motricity 103–131
Hypnic physiologic myoclonias 70

Ibotenic acid, thalamic nucleus 73, 74
Imperative stimulus 77
Input-output linkage 6
Interface to environment 53, 54
Interference by brain stimulus 99, 100
Intracortical microstimulation, finger
  movements 33–37
Intraspinal branching 6
Involuntary muscle activation 93, 94
Ipsilateral corticobulbar supply 96–98
Ipsilateral pathway 14

Joint movements, paraplegics 58–60
Jung, Richard 121

Kennard principle 116
Kinematic synergies 47–50
Kinematography 121–127
Knee
  extensor movement 54, 55
  markers 48

Laboratory reflexes 117
Lashley, Karl Spencer 124, 125
Latency shortening 93
Lateral reticular nucleus 6
Leg
  extensor muscles 61, 62
  flexor muscles 61
  movements, rhythm generation 114
  muscle activation 59
Lidocaine, SMA inactivation 35–40
Limb
  configuration, grasping 28–30
  muscles 96

Load
   force 26
   receptors 47
Locomotor training, paraplegics
   57–64
Locus coeruleus neurons 70

M1 motor cortex area 82
   precision grip 33–42
Magnetic pulses over the scalp 91
Magnetic resonance imaging 14
Masticatory muscles 96
Microgravity, equilibrium 48, 50
Monkeys
   grip patterns 20, 21
   precision grip 33–42
Monosynaptic nature, reflexes 105
Motoneuron pool 105
Motor activity, sleep 65–74
Motor behavior
   measurement 13
   neuronal activity 6, 7
Motor control 10–12
Motor cortex 2, 6, 8
   hand movements 33–42
   neurons 7
   pyramidal tract 2
   readiness potential 81
Motor deficits 4–7
Motor disorders during sleep 71–73
Motor equivalence 121–127
Motor evoked responses 92–101
Motor invariance 11, 12
Motor preparedness 107
Motor reorganization 14
Motor schemas 22
Movement
   analysis 52–56
   coordination 108–112
   duration during grasping 30
   parameters 7
   rhythmic 112–115
   time 27, 28
Muscle
   afferents 6
   atonia during sleep 66–70
   field 6
   lengthening and shortening 61
   tone 105
Myoclonias, thalamus 73, 74
Myoclonic jerks 70, 73, 74

Neurology, motor control 115–119
Neuronal activity
   during sleep 66

motor behavior 6, 7
   recording 13, 14
Neuronal correlates, movement 10–12
Neurons
   discharge 8, 9
   pragmatic processing 22
   rhythmic discharges 114, 115
Newborn stepping 57
Night acroparesthesia 66
Nocturnal myoclonus 72
Nocturnal paroxysmal dystonia 72, 73
Non-REM sleep 65, 67, 71
   sleep disorders 72, 73

Object attributes, grasping 22–27
Object orientation 25, 26
   limb configuration 28–30
Object size
   grip patterns 23–25
   timing of grip 28
Oculomotor system 100
Opposition space 28–30
Optoelectronic systems, movement
   analysis 53–56

P wave 69
Parallel activation, movements 27, 28
Parallel organization 14
Paraplegics, locomotor training 57–64
Parasomnias 71–73
Parietal cortex, pragmatic processing 22
Parkinson's disease, reaction time 120
PET scans 130, 131
Phasic events 86, 87
Physiology of motor control 104–115
Plasticity of brain 97, 98
Polysynaptic flexion reflex 67
Pontine neurons 67
Postcontraction phenomenon 93–95
Posterior intralaminar thalamus, myoclonias 73,
   74
Post-second stimulus 88, 89
Postural adjustments 44–50, 105–107
Postural anticipation 105–107
Postural shifts during sleep 65, 66
Posture 105, 106
   volitional and movement
      coordination 108–112
Power grip 20
Pragmatic processing 22
Prazosin, locomotor activity 62
Precision grip 5, 7, 8, 20–23
   monkeys 33–42
Prehensile activity 19, 20
Premotor cortex 10

Premotor positivity 77
Preshaping the hand 23, 24
Pre-SMA 37
Primary motor cortical areas, precision
  grip 33–42
Primates, grip patterns 20, 21
Principle of equal simplicity 124, 126
Pronation 25, 26
Proximal limb muscles 97
Psychological aspects, motor control 119–127
Push-pull movement 11
Pyramidal syndrome 3, 116
Pyramidal tract
  history 1–7
  neurons 3, 6, 7
    during sleep 66, 67
    rhythmic discharges 115
  origin 8–12
Pyramidotomy 3

Raphe neurons 70
Reaching 12, 27–30
Reaction time paradigm 119, 120
Readiness potential 77, 79–86, 120, 121
  spatial distribution 88, 89
Reflex
  depression 67–70
  studies 104, 105
Reflexes during sleep 67–70
Relayed pyramidal discharge 3
REM sleep 65–74
  behavior disorder 71
Restless legs syndrome 71, 72
Rhythm generation 112–116
Rhythms, hand movement 87

S1-S2 stimulation paradigm 81–83
Saccades, direct 100
Saturday evening paralysis 66
Scaling, subjective 24, 25
Scalp 88
Single action current 112
Sleep, motor activity 65–74
Sleepwalking 71
Slow cortical potentials 77–89
SMA-L, SMA-R, see Supplementary motor area
Spasticity 3, 115, 116
  paraplegics 59
Sphincter muscle 96
Spinal cord, spinal circuits 105
Spinal locomotor activity 57–64
Spinal motoneurons 92
Stance phase, walking 54, 55, 62
Stepping movements 57–59
Stimulus spread in brain 95

Stretch reflex 116, 117
Supplementary motor area 7, 8, 88
  ablation 41
  bimanual coordination 12
  discovery 117–119
  inactivation 33–42
  neuronal activity 10, 11
  precision grip 33–42
  readiness potential 81
  surgical lesions 40, 41
Swing phase, walking 62

Tactile-motor loops 27
Task difficulty, movement 28
Temporal invariance, grasping 28
Thalamus, sleep regulation 73, 74
Thumb, opposable 20
Tibialis anterior muscle, locomotion 60–63
Tonic activity, neurons 107, 108
Tonogenic centers, brainstem 107
Tool use behavior 20
Tooth grinding 73
Touch 19
Trajectories of limb, grasping 28–30
Transcallosal inhibition 98, 99
Transcortical reflexes 6
Transcranial magnetic stimulation 91–101
Transneuronal labelling 9
Tridimensional movement 10
Trochanter markers 48
Trunk bending movements 45, 46

Upper trunk bending, center of gravity 45–47

Ventral horn neurons 66, 67
Visual evoked potentials 81–83, 85
Visuomotor channels 27
  separate 30
Visuomotor transformation 19, 22–25,
  28
Vogt, Cécile 117–119
Vogt, Oskar 117–119
Voluntary movement
  coordination 108–112
  pyramidal tract 2, 3
  self-paced 77–89
Voluntary muscle activation 93, 94

Wachholder, Kurt 108–112
Walking, analysis 54, 55
Warning stimulus 77
Wrist
  extension 110, 111
  flexion 110, 111
  rotation 25, 26, 30